Tales of a
Gluten-Free Gypsy

Tales of a Gluten-Free Gypsy

by Judith Fine-Sarchielli

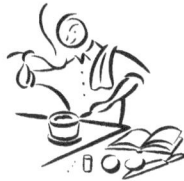

Highly Sensitive People
PUBLICATIONS

Tales of a Gluten-Free Gypsy
© 2014 Judith Fine-Sarchielli
Photographs and illustrations copyright to their respective creators as noted

Published by HighlySensitivePeople®, 750 West 15th Ave., Escondido, CA 92025

ISBN 978-0-9824808-3-0

Printed and bound in the United States of America

First Printing — July 2014

Tales of a Gluten-Free Gypsy has been published for informational and entertainment purposes only, and is not intended to replace or substitute for any professional therapy, medical diagnosis, health practice, treatment, nutritional or other advice. The suggestions, statements and recipes presented herein are drawn from the experiences of the author and represent personal opinions, and are not intended as medical advice for specific diagnoses, medical conditions or making any evaluation as to the risks and benefits of a particular health or dietary protocol. Before incorporating any of the information presented in this book into practice or embarking upon any diet or nutritional regime, the publisher encourages you to consult with a medical professional or licensed health care provider.

Cover design by Jim Hallowes, publisher; book design, layout and production by Edward Rapka. Typeset in Goudy and Bitstream Vera Sans, with headings in Corbel Bold. Photo credits: Cover and page 14 (anguskirk, flickr.com/foter.com, used under Creative Commons license); pages 20, 46, 56, 94, 112, 124, 132 (Dreamstime.com); 69 (Dr. Peter Osborne, Gluten-FreeSociety.org); 74 (E. Maza, Maza Studios, used with permission); 103 (user J.J., Wikipedia.org, Creative Commons license); 115 (City of Denver); 175 (© Andy F., Creative Commons license). See https://creativecommons.org/licenses/by-nc-nd/2.0/legalcode.

Dedication

My inspiration throughout the last two years (of four years) as I wrote Tales has been my granddaughter, Bianca, who is almost three years old. Her joy for life, love for me and her family, spontaneity, and integrity have given me the energy to move through the many editing and other publishing challenges I experienced.

I hope to share this book with her when she is older and understands how important she is to my life and creativity. All the meals her Florentine great-grandmother, Bianca, handed down to me I made for little Bianca over the many months while babysitting her 25-plus hours a week. I wrote them with the gluten-free lifestyle in mind that I hope she will incorporate when she understands the importance of a healthy diet and lifestyle.

Acknowledgements

As I wrote my cookbook-memoir, *Tales of A Gluten-Free Gypsy*, my caravan ride was a wild one, with many jolts and unexpected turns. I hung on for dear life through the long journey and look forward my readers' feedback. I want my readers to understand that in the last five years, much has been discovered about the gluten issue and the experts have clarified the difference between Celiac Disease and gluten-sensitivity after for the first time in history. Non-Celiac Disease Sensitivity, (NCDS), is actually more rampant than Celiac disease. I am gluten-sensitive (NCGS), and owe my life to what I have uncovered about gluten and grains.

I wrote *Tales* to warn people that the gluten-free diet fad is very dangerous and can lead to a variety of fatal diseases. It is essential that anyone who attempts this gluten-free diet works with a gluten specialist or does the trial I suggest in the book. More accurate tests have been developed in the last few years, but false negatives still abound, and there is not one blood test for gluten sensitivity that is 100% accurate at this time.

I also want my readers to know that my twenty years in Italy was priceless for me as an actress, artist and designer, and enabled me to have a career as a chef, wife and mother in Italy and the U.S. while I raised my son. Bianca Sarchielli was my Florentine mother-in-law—a Zen-style master cooking teacher who taught me to cook and shared authentic recipes from the Tuscan tradition that are hundreds of years old.

There will never be enough special words to express my gratitude to my team: my publisher Jim Hallowes (*www.highlysensitivepeople.com*), Edward Rapka, the brilliant designer who was patient beyond belief with my numerous drafts, and Kathy Vilim, my copy editor, who was loyal and a talented detective who wove her way through the maze of my gypsy life. Kathy jumped on my caravan as copy editor after the first galley proof edits and was immediately faced with many technological challenges that she overcame with an astute eye, an open mind, grace, and professionalism.

In addition, Bernard Selling, my surrogate agent and popular author of historical novels, was there with wise advice and my lawyer Gerry Bryant (*www.calawyersfor-thearts.org*) helped me focus and stay on the path to complete my book.

Thanks also to Maria Hill, Steve Kirchner, Diane Sukiennek, Suzanne Weirich and Jean Uckurt, who read preliminary chapters, for their generosity, valuable suggestions, and encouragement. This team has seen me through all the unexpected challenges, both technological and emotional, over the six years it has taken me to write and publish my book.

I was able to stay the course on my *Tales* travels due to all the support and love I received from brother Doug, son Sacha, ex-husband Massimo (with whom I realized my dream to become a true gypsy, and who gypsied his way to the other side three years ago), past and present life coaches, therapists, teachers, gurus, lovers and fellow gypsies I met and adventured with in my caravan, as I moved along the diverse paths of my often impulsive and open-road travels.

Many exciting and synchronistic, fleeting moments as I focused on this book showed me I was on the right path as far as the topic. Many times, strangers and I have shared in-depth information about my and my G-F community's feelings and thoughts about the gluten-free diet fad. As a marketing coach for creative entrepreneurs, I start my clients out with diet information and focus on gluten. I encourage entrepreneurs and creatives to build on a healthy platform to bring their ideas to the world and help save the planet.

I promise you a true adventure and better health for you, your family and friends, with the information you will learn when you join my gluten-free gypsy caravan as you travel with me on my life's journey!

EAT REAL!

THE JOURNEY…

FOREWORD

I first met Judith Fine-Sarchielli while serving as director of The WANT® Institute, the non-profit educational organization founded by the noted relationship counselor, author and Highly Sensitive Person (HSP) Dr. Pat Allen. HSPs comprise 15–20% of the population and process incoming information and subtleties in their environment more deeply than the average person. As a student of the Institute for over three years who graduated to become a Certified Communications Educator, Judith epitomized to me both the ideal student and the major traits of an HSP: bright, attentive, curious, tenacious, and passionate about learning Dr. Pat Allen's valuable communication information.

When Judith volunteered to give a valuable presentation about gluten sensitivity to Institute students, I became even more impressed, especially with her expertise on how gluten affects highly sensitive persons as well as the general public, and realized the importance of the issue of gluten and the gluten-free diet to HSPs. I immediately suggested that she put her information into more comprehensive form as a book we could publish.

It's my privilege to finally be publishing that very book, outlining the pros and cons of the gluten-free diet and stressing the fact that it should be viewed as something more than a fad, along with Judith's fascinating personal stories of how she gypsied her way across the U.S. and Europe. In today's society with many people struggling with overweight and diabetes becoming epidemic, Judith's mind-opening cookbook-memoir, *Tales of a Gluten-Free Gypsy*, will stir up a controversial debate as regards the "Ideal Diet"—especially now that the FDA is revising their outdated Diet Pyramid that has been held up for many years as a nutritional bellwether for the North American public.

Judith's aim is to educate about the misinformation on gluten and help set the record straight. Even in today's health-conscious climate, few doctors and nutritionists have the whole story about celiac disease and gluten sensitivity. Judith explains where a gluten-free diet can make an important contribution to one's health, and also how as a fad this diet can potentially harm many people, HSP and non-HSP alike.

This informative, well-researched and documented book weaves vital facts about gluten and diet in an enticing and, pardon the expression, "delicious" way. Judith pulls no punches as she educates as well as entertains you. As you'll soon discover, she is passionate about the welfare of others. She has also provided an entire section of resources that will facilitate the reader in doing more research on health topics in addition to that of the gluten issue.

I cannot think of a single person more qualified to write this book. Judith lived in Tuscany for 20 years and has had careers as a gluten-free Tuscan-style chef, cooking instructor, nutritional consultant and author. She cares deeply about people, and in addition to her Institute certification holds certifications as both a Vision Board Consultant and a Transactional Analysis Practitioner. Typical of her HSP trait, Judith is also an intuitive and vibrational educator, communications strategist, and marketing coach for creative entrepreneurs.

I've often lectured about the defining characteristics of Highly Sensitive Persons which include being very creative, having a deep appreciation for art, nature and music, kind of "addicted to learning," striving to be perfect themselves and championing a belief in universal justice. With their gifts, however, comes a downside as HSPs can often get overwhelmed and need frequent "alone time" to keep their passions in balance. All these characteristics, as you'll read, apply to Judith!

Sometimes HSPs are also called *alphas*, those people who are in touch with both their masculine and feminine energies, and often face an on-going tug of war between their head and heart. These creative and unique people often feel like outsiders. They have to make an extra effort to fit into society, and often feel like gypsies or that they are "from another planet!"

One of my popular talks focuses on celebrities I believe qualify as HSPs, an illustrious group that ranges across Carl Jüng, Albert Einstein, Emily Dickinson, Abraham Lincoln, Leonardo Da Vinci, Georgia O'Keefe, Howard Hughes, Jane Goodall, Edgar Allen Poe, Princess Diana, Walt Disney, it seems most all comedians from Woody Allen and Steve Martin to Andy Kaufman and Jim Carrey, and of course many, many musicians from Mozart and Beethoven to Bob Dylan and Barbara Streisand. It is perhaps best epitomized by the late Apple Computer founder, Steve Jobs, who summed-up the influence of HSPs:

> "The ones who are crazy enough to think that they can change the world, are the ones who do."

His view is similar to a wonderful quote by famed anthropologist Margaret Mead, who said:

> "Never doubt that a small group of thoughtful, committed citizens can change the world; indeed, it's the only thing that ever has."

As you may have already noticed, I like quotes! So, with that being said, here's an observation that many visitors to the Highly Sensitive People website say resonates with them, and I think it pretty well sums up the nature of an HSP. It's from Pearl S. Buck, recipient of the Pulitzer Prize and the Nobel Prize in Literature:

> "The truly creative mind in any field is no more than this:
> A human creature born abnormally, inhumanly sensitive.
> To him...
> > a touch is a blow,
> > a sound is a noise,
> > a misfortune is a tragedy,
> > a joy is an ecstasy,
> > a friend is a lover,
> > a lover is a god,
> > and failure is death.
> Add to this cruelly delicate organism the overpowering necessity to create, create, create — so that without the creating of music or poetry or books or buildings or something of meaning, his very breath is cut off from him. He must create, must pour out creation. By some strange, unknown, inward urgency he is not really alive unless he is creating."

It's not surprising then that, as an HSP, Judith has joined a grassroots movement to change the way people look at the industrialization of our food chain. And because of Judith's passion about this important topic and her "overpowering necessity" to create and help heal the planet I can now invite you to start on an exciting journey as my dear friend Judith Fine-Sarchielli spins her tales as a gluten-free gypsy dedicated to exploring the mysteries of the perfect diet for herself and her readers!

Jim Hallowes
Founder of Highly Sensitive People®
and *www.HighlySensitivePeople.com*
Los Angeles, California, June 2014

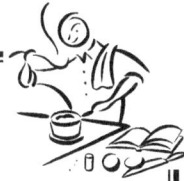

INTRODUCTION
FROM AUTHOR TO READER

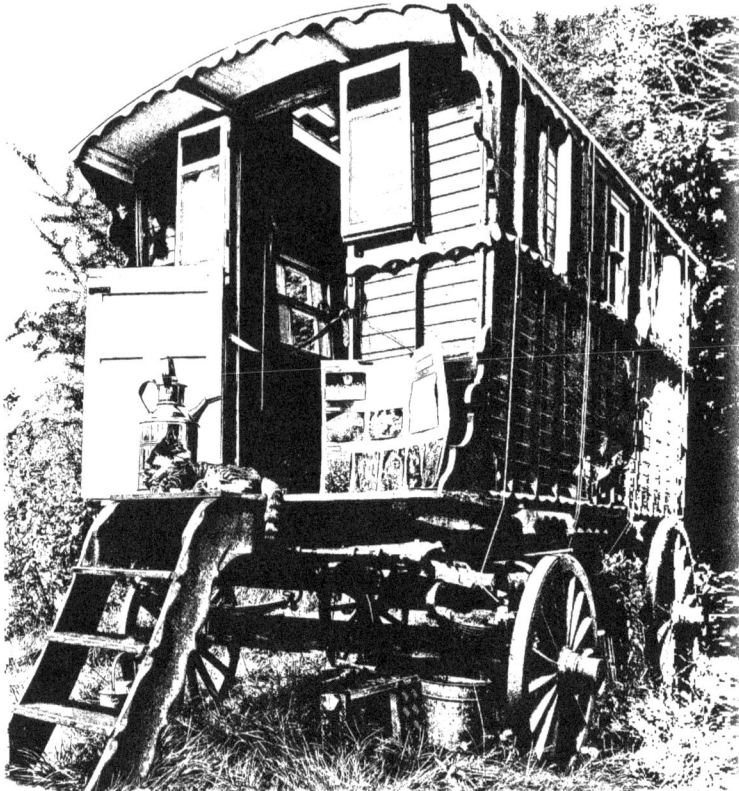

"MAY THIS FOOD BE BEFORE YOU,
AND IN YOUR MEMORY,
AND MAY IT PROFIT US
IN GOOD HEALTH AND IN GOOD SPIRIT."

(Ancient Gypsy proverb)

I often ask myself, "How did I ever end up becoming an 'almost' Tuscan, an Italian citizen, and the mother of a bi-cultural son who was blessed by Jackie Kennedy at birth with a dual citizenship?" And how did I discover that I was gluten-sensitive and a Highly Sensitive Person (HSP)? My answers are in these tales of a gluten-free gypsy who discovered her essence in her mid-seventies after digging deep along her gypsy caravan path.

In my mid-seventies, I discovered that I was gluten-sensitive and an HSP. I wrote this book because, until recently, I always felt outside of society. I believed that I was an "eccentric and a kook," because that's what people labeled me. My mother called me crazy in the midst of our emotional battles as a teenager, and I believed her. I have changed these labels to "Creative" and "Evolutionary Leader." This book is targeted to both the gluten-sensitive and the Highly Sensitive Person (HSP), those who are more vulnerable to food, diet, and most everything else, rather than the other 80% of the world's population. HSP, the psychological category that is hereditary, has been re-labeled in the DSM IV (*Diagnostic and Statistical Manual of Mental Disorders*) from "Over Sensitive" to "Highly Sensitive."

I am a well-informed nutritional researcher, author, and inspired marketing coach for creative Baby Boomer entrepreneurs. Although I am not a doctor or certified nutritionist, I often have more cutting-edge information about diet at my fingertips than do many health care professionals, because I have spent most of the last thirty years in nutritional research for myself and my entrepreneurial marketing clients.

As a Highly Sensitive Child, I wanted to heal the world. Today, as an adult HSP, I created this cookbook-memoir as part of my mission to leave a legacy of valuable diet and health information as I continue to assist and inspire others who face dietary and nutritional challenges. I hope to inspire people and educate them so that they, too, can experience the joys of gourmet meals without deprivation. With the knowledge you gain from this book, you can also be a "gluten-free gypsy" open to new and inspiring food adventures. You will be happier, healthier, and more alive when you learn to EAT REAL!

Gluten sensitivity, intolerance, low energy reserves, and Celiac Disease (CD) are challenges that affect both the HSP and the general population in many ways. The numbers of people with health issues increase daily because, in a changing global environment, our diet is radically altered due to food industrialization, environmental and chemical toxins, and stress. I urge you not to treat gluten intolerance, gluten sensitivity, or Celiac Disease as a fad. The current fad, sponsored by major corporations, industries and government, is dangerous. It is essential to understand the facts if one is gluten-sensitive, gluten-intolerant (allergic), or Celiac. Gluten sensitivity often leads to CD, and potentially to other diseases, and terminal illness. If you are truly affected by gluten, the experts advise to test as soon as possible or do an elimination diet to remove all gluten from your diet.

I want this book to educate and inform gluten-sensitives and HSPs about living gluten-free while maintaining the possibilities of enjoying delicious food. My gluten-free platform and program for the general public is not a fad. It is a lifestyle that can inspire you, your family, and friends.

When I was an eight-year-old child in Denver, Colorado, I discovered Europe through my aunt's art books. Denver was too small for my imagination, and my hunger for Europe grew more compelling as I went from childhood to teens. At age 17 as a Fine Arts major in college, I studied the lives and art of the Renaissance masters I had read about in those childhood forays into a book about famous artists' lives. I was obsessed with a desire to see the real thing and badgered my parents until they finally relented and sent me to Paris to study French and painting. (I lied to them and said I was going to be an au pair with a French family.)

My adventures began as I left the stifling 1950s mid-America as a naive 18-year-old, and sailed for Europe to meet my prince. I found a romantic little attic room in a pension on the Left Bank of Paris and went to Florence on a side trip from my art school in Paris. I met Massimo, my destiny and Gypsy Prince on the Ponte Vecchio ("Old Bridge") where Dante first saw his mentor and inspiration for *The Divine Comedy*, Beatrice. She inspired him to write the book that would revolutionize the Italian language and define the modern

Renaissance philosophy I was convinced that I had met my soul mate. I ended up living with and then marrying my gypsy prince and learned to cook traditional, centuries-old Tuscan recipes from my mother-in-law, Bianca.

Gluten-sensitivity, gluten intolerance, and Celiac Disease (an immune reaction to eating the protein gluten) are far more than an occasional tummy upset. Mayo Clinic research suggests that Celiac Disease has become a major public health issue. According to Mayo studies, undiagnosed Celiac Disease can quadruple the risk of death. Mayo researchers learned that those whose gluten intolerance had not been diagnosed in the 1950s were four times likelier to have died. "Having undiagnosed Celiac Disease is not good for you," Dr. Murray of the Mayo Clinic, warns. "It may take 20 to 30 years for that risk to become apparent. But there's a good chance it's a problem." Mayo researchers are working to discover the causes and improve diagnosis.

http://discoverysedge.mayo.edu/celiac-disease/index.cfm

THE IMPACT OF GLUTEN SENSITIVITY
Between 5% and 10% of all people may suffer from a gluten sensitivity of some form
1 out of every 100 has Celiac Disease (CD)
97% of Americans estimated to have Celiac Disease are not diagnosed
Celiac Disease has over 300 known symptoms
30% of the U.S. population is estimated to have the genes necessary for Celiac Disease
There are currently 0 drugs available to treat Celiac Disease
Gluten-free (GF) foods are, on average, 242% more expensive than their non-GF counterparts
The U.S. Department of Agriculture projects that the gluten-free industries' revenues will reach more than $2.0 Billion by 2012
People with Celiac Disease dine out 80% less than they used to before diagnosis and believe less that only 10% of eating establishments have a "very good" or "good" understanding of Gluten-Free diets
The average cost of a misdiagnosis is $5,000 – $12,000 per person per year
Celiac Disease is a hereditary condition. If you have Celiac Disease, you can expect that 4–12% of your first-degree relatives will also have the condition
60% of children and 41% of adults diagnosed during the study were asymptomatic
Statistic Verification Data from www.statistics.com Source: National Institutes of Health, Univ. of Chicago Celiac Disease Center Date Verified: 3.19.2012

As a food consultant at Whole Foods Market in 2005, I was not surprised to learn that, at that time, most Americans were ignorant about the danger of the gluten-free fad. Most people didn't even know about gluten! The Celiac Organization *(www.celiac.org)* reports that one-percent (1%) of the North American population is affected with CD. This is an alarming 1 in every 100 people, and the numbers are rapidly increasing. Ninety-percent of people who have gluten challenges are unaware of this potentially dangerous problem.

My promise to you is that if you find you test for gluten issues and are consistent with your authentic gluten-free eating habits, you will notice improvement immediately. Opinions differ about a final cure; however, if you are gluten-intolerant or sensitive and not a full-blown celiac, you can be almost symptom-free in nine months or less if you hold to the Celiac Disease (CD) dietary rules. My readers will learn new information about how gluten increases sensitivity on all levels and the steps to take to make life less stressful.

Because I follow an authentic gluten-free (grain and sugar-free) and Paleo regime (increased vegetables, animal protein, and fats), my life is now more enjoyable and richer in every way. I regulate my eating habits and lifestyle and avoid triggers that used to challenge my full participation in all of what this life has to offer.

Many of the classic Tuscan recipes in my book are centuries old. As a Tuscan chef, I have pleased my clients' palates with them for over thirty years. In this book, I have adapted these timeless recipes to suit the gluten-free and Paleo lifestyle. I hope they will become part of your family's and friends' traditions for many generations to come. I have presented these recipes in the form of a traditional Italian menu: *Antipasto* (Appetizer), *Primo Piatto* (First Course), *Contorno* (Side Dish), and *Dolce* (Dessert). These are recipes that appeal to the gypsy in us all, as they are both appetizing and nutritious.

The old Tuscan saying, "Cook like a peasant and eat like royalty" can still ring true today.

1

JUMP ON THE GYPSY WAGON WITH ME!

THE APPETIZER

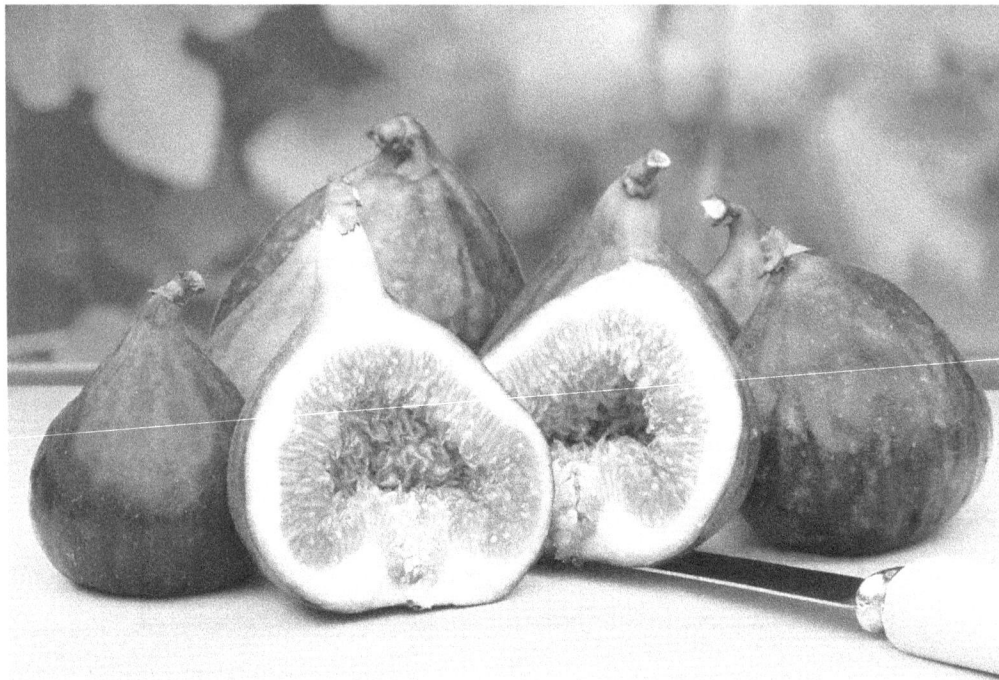

ANTIPASTO

This tapenade is a classic and delicious for any occasion, especially for picnics. You can use it instead of mayonnaise or mustard to perk up raw vegetables or spread on apple slices. I always have some in the fridge and serve it as an antipasto for unexpected guest snacks or dinner parties. All nuts and seeds should be soaked to bring out their essential vitality.

FIG and WALNUT TAPENADE

SERVES 8

INGREDIENTS

1 cup dried figs
½ cup organic apple juice
1 cup walnuts, soaked and dried
1 Tbsp. organic olive oil
½ teaspoon balsamic vinegar
1 Tbsp. fresh rosemary leaves, minced

PREPARATION

Process figs for 30 seconds, until well chopped

Add apple juice and pulse to create a paste

Add walnuts and pulse until incorporated

Add olive oil, vinegar, and rosemary and pulse again
for 30 seconds until smooth

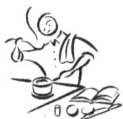

Chef's Note

You can choose to make the tapenade paste chunky or smooth depending on how much you process it at each step. Add an anchovy to the mix for a deeper flavor.

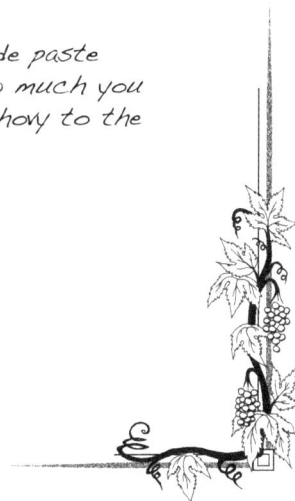

*T*he prophet Abraham held an open house and fed people all through the day as a ploy to educate them about the Teachings, a very clever idea to attract his guests and to share his wisdom. At the same time, he also reminded them that God blessed both Abraham and his guests. Not everyone is a philosopher or wants to learn new ideas, but everyone likes to eat, especially when it's free. The question is—what do we eat and how does food affect us on physical, mental, and spiritual levels? And even more important, what nourishes our brains?

Yummm! My stomach growls and my mouth waters. I look with delight and anticipation at the appetizer on my dinner plate. My table is laid with fresh flowers, and a candle flickers in the breeze. I am gazing at the red, purple, and pink sunset from the tree house-like studio where I live and work in the hills of Topanga Canyon, California. Tonight's menu consists of customized, authentic, and delicious Tuscan recipes that I have transformed to gluten-free. I am grateful that I can enjoy my meal for something more than the look and taste. After many years of searching for the perfect lifestyle diet, I have finally reached the point where enjoyment will not lead to suffering stomach pains and mood swings immediately afterwards. Dining has become a pleasure that I look forward to each evening with delight and have no gluten after-effects. I love to EAT REAL!

I had an indelible dream when I was just eight-years-old which inspired me to create this cookbook now in my mid-seventies. As a Highly Sensitive Child (HSP) I wanted to heal the world. Today, as an adult HSP, my mission is to leave a legacy of integrity as I continue to assist and inspire others who face dietary and nutritional challenges. I hope to influence people and educate them to know that they, too, can experience the joys of eating gourmet meals without feeling deprived. With the knowledge you gain from this book, you will also be a "gluten-free gypsy," open to new and fulfilling food adventures.

Even the most simple meal connects us to people around the planet we will never know who grow and manufacture our daily food. We are connected because of our basic need to connect to our family and friends through the meals we share and even what we eat on the run. You will be happier, healthier, and more alive when you choose your foods as well as how you eat, where you eat, and who you eat with. You will EAT REAL! for a longer and healthier life.

I am an expert nutritional researcher, author, and marketing coach for creative baby boomer entrepreneurs, not a doctor or nutritionist. I find that I often have more cutting-edge information about diet at my fingertips than do many certified professionals, because I have spent most days researching and coaching about nutrition for the last six years. It has taken me decades of eating, experimenting and researching with my own diet to understand my challenges and now I can relax and enjoy my food as an integrated part of my life.

When I began to investigate my diet as a gluten-free gypsy, my brain was consumed with research, multi-cognition tasking, rumination, and experimentation. I clarified which foods enhanced my overall being and gave me the most value for my time and energy on a daily basis. While I was healing, I was grateful to have healthy food to eat, but I didn't always enjoy it, and was often hungry and bored with my diet because I didn't know how to balance my nutritional intake.

Even though I tried a wide variety of diets over the years with some intermittent success: Mediterranean, Blood Type, Low-Carbohydrate, Vegetarian, Macrobiotic, Yeast-free, and Raw, still I experienced frequent gut and emotional pain.

For thirty years living with, and then married to, my Florentine husband, I dined in Italy, Paris, London, other parts of Western Europe, New York City and San Francisco. Now, as an older woman living in LA and a newbie to the gluten issue, I had to reconsider my diet again. I wanted to celebrate the seeds I planted as a child and the fruition and blossoming of those seeds that resulted in my increased well-being.

Now, I am no longer anxious and fearful about which foods to eat. I have finally found a regime and nutritional balance that always works for me. I am excited to share this information and some of these recipes with you. I want you to feel the same passion I did when I chose this regime and committed to it. I want you to feel encouraged to inspire your family and friends and then rejoice in their well-being together.

Only recently, as a gluten-sensitive HSP, have I been able to put the exact words around who I am, because now I think with more clarity when I eat right. The brain is our first digestive organ and is influenced by our senses.

Today, I no longer experience "foggy brain syndrome"— the result of years of eating around my food allergies and cancer treatments. Instead, I feel freedom and joy. And what I eat is one of the essential components of my essence and core foundation.

I EAT REAL.

I have gobbled up seventy-seven years' worth of foods from different cultures as I "gypsyed" my way through the menus and delicacies of the United States and Europe. In the past seven years, my G-F–HSP gypsy caravan was my shopping cart as I traveled from farmers' markets to specialty food stores, healthy food and ethnic markets, and mom-and-pop grocery stores. I have spent thousands of hours over the years reading labels, as I searched for authentic gluten-free product discoveries, only to find that most of the "gluten-free" products I found were *not* authentic gluten-free.

Have you been a gluten-free gypsy as you wander around gluten-free information, diets, and grocery stores searching for the right foods to satisfy your palate and your nutritional needs? Do you still hunt for the right food for your perfect diet? Are you still confused by your choices? Do you know what foods are truly true gluten-free? Do you read label details on processed foods? Do you call and question manufacturers or producers and talk to store managers about what does and doesn't work for you with their products and services? Do they answer your requests with an open and willing attitude?

Several years ago, when I was a food consultant at the Whole Foods market in the San Fernando Valley of California, I suggested to the store manager that they invest in some gluten-free products, as we had a growing number of customers that were sensitive to wheat. He did not seem to hear me then. Today, however, they have hundreds of G-F products, which bring in billions of dollars a year. Today, even the supermarkets have begun to compete for this market with organic produce and other g-f products.

Did you know that most "gluten-free" products on the store shelves now are *not* G-F? Even an infinitesimal amount of gluten can cause you to be glutened and sick. The FDA label rulings regarding "gluten-free" product ingredients are too low and not accurate. Gluten-free has become a popular, dangerous fad because the ingredients in these "gluten-free" products are loaded with cross-grains, GMO and sugar, which can be potentially harmful.

This book teaches my readers how to EAT REAL. You can create your own garden of paradise where you can enjoy the fruits of the seeds you plant.

As a young HSP child, a teen and into late adulthood, I was always frustrated with my dietary issues—allergies to wheat, soy, corn, nuts, and dairy. I always wanted to satisfy my palate and be symptom-free. In my late sixties, I learned that I was gluten-intolerant, which changed the way I looked at food forever. I felt frustrated and depressed that many of my favorite foods were now off limits. At first it was suggested that I was a celiac. To this day, I still have never done a gluten analysis or biopsy. At the beginning of my HSP G-F journey, and after several years of experimentation and research, I found that the elimination diet worked for me; I eliminated all gluten products and cross-grains from my diet for two weeks and then added them back for one day. That day, I had all of the negative symptoms which I had researched and had experienced in the past, which I discuss in Chapter Four.

When I was eight years old, I dreamt that I could heal the world's pain. I was too young to heal my own pain, so instead I projected my desire to heal my physical and psychological pain on healing humanity. This was a big goal for a little girl, but I stand by that goal to this day. From early adolescence, frustration and depression led to increased mood swings and frequent suicidal thoughts. I was hypersensitive and emotionally reactive, overly anxious, and had problems with impulse control. All of that changed when I learned about gluten and high sensitivity. Statistics show that women have a higher incidence of gluten challenges and high sensitivity than men, and more gluten-sensitivity as well.

In my early forties, I was diagnosed with breast cancer and followed the classic protocol of the time: mastectomy, chemotherapy, radiation, and post-surgery medications. The chemicals in the medications almost destroyed my pancreas. With the help of alternative medicine, especially Chinese acupuncture and herbs, psychological counseling, yoga, and self-help studies, I began to heal my emotional inner self, as well as my physical self. Perhaps my childhood dream could manifest. But how could I heal the world if I wasn't whole?

As a small child, I always followed my grandfather's lead about new food and flavors. Thanks to my love for him, my palate is still inspired by curiosity about food, and now as the grandmother of a toddler, I want to help develop my three-year-old baby granddaughter, Bianca's, palate so she will grow up to have a similar enjoyment and curiosity. (Italian babies eat everything their family eats with appetite and delight.)

What did you eat today? Did you choose or take what was fastest or cheapest? How did you eat and with whom did you eat? Were you angry or happy when you cooked your meal? What and how we eat affects much more than our own physical, mental, and spiritual self. Our food choices affect, and are affected by, economics, social structure, commerce, nature, history, health, the environment, animals, and people all around the planet.

I incorporated the "Know Thyself" teachings from the Bible as I explored my inner self through therapy and self-help books. I learned that the stomach is a second brain, and digestion is influenced by many diverse factors. Feelings, emotions, and moods are connected to the gut. For almost fifty years, my gut was so compromised from allergies and gluten sensitivity that I had lost my "gut instincts" and became involved with many negative people and situations. The "Me in Me" was out of control and lost until I learned about gluten and began to regain control of my life.

In the meantime, from the age of 18, I rocketed through eight different schools, colleges, and universities until I got my BFA, as well as several jobs in Manhattan, where I continued to study for my MA in art history. Then I started to learn about computers, and that is another story.

As a rebellious teenager, my mother often yelled, "You're crazy!" whenever we argued, which was often. I would beg her to send me to a therapist. In the 1950s, that would have been a social disgrace for our family. In the early 1970s when I lived in Italy, I looked for an Italian therapist with no results. When I returned to the U.S. in 1974, I began to work with a Gestalt therapy group and gypsyed my way through several different therapeutic styles up until 2011. My last therapist, Sharon Dunas, was the most effective, because she understood my need for self-expression and was a true healer. Sharon helped me see my future career and relationship potential as she helped me clean the fog of depression from my crystal ball.

In an early therapy session with Sharon, I remembered that my passion for food began as a three-year-old, when I sneaked to the refrigerator for cod liver oil in the middle of the night. One time my father caught me and was very angry to find me looking for cod liver oil in the refrigerator in my pajamas.

I received the only threat and punishment of my life from him at that time. As a child and now, I have always loved to eat — the more exotic the food, the better.

I dined on raw oysters with my beloved Grandpa Sam on Sundays at Denver's finest hotel, The Brown Palace, when I was four years old. We would carefully choose all of Grandpa Sam's favorite delicacies: smoked salmon, caviar, roast beef, smoked Rainbow trout, and his very favorite — oysters on the half shell. Everything was displayed on huge banquet tables with elaborate ice sculptures and beautiful flower arrangements. We even had flowers and a candle on our table, though it was still daylight. I was fascinated and enjoyed all the different looks, tastes, and textures of these exotic foods. Of everything on my plate, I loved the oysters the most.

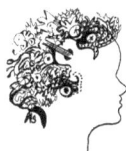

"Don't chew, just swallow!"
His dark eyes twinkled as he commanded me with his gruff Russian voice. He had grown up as the ninth son of a teacher of Rabbis. Because his family depended on the community for sustenance, as a child Grandpa Sam would cheat on the orthodox kosher diet and sneak oysters from the Black Sea, which he secretly gobbled up, never feeling guilty with these indulgences because he was starving. His black eyes sparkled as we enjoyed them together. This is one of my first memories of joy that was connected to food.

In the tiny canyon in the Santa Monica Mountains near Los Angeles where I live there is a Mexican restaurant, a gourmet food shop, a pizzeria, two cafes, one tiny raw food place, an expensive French/California-style bistro, and a very expensive, touristy, gourmet healthy food restaurant with a prize-winning list of organic wines and a couple of gluten-free items on the menu. It's hard to find any good gluten-free restaurants here or in the nearest town, which is

15 minutes away, except for a few small restaurants and pizzerias that serve G-F pizzas. I sometimes take my three-year-old granddaughter, Bianca, to a gourmet gluten-free restaurant in Topanga. She loves sweet potato fries!

In this small community I know several gluten-free residents. Many others here, as well as all over the world, experience digestive and mood swing problems as they age and struggle with new and increased allergies, gluten intolerance, obesity, diabetes, alcoholism, Fibromyalgia, Chronic Fatigue Syndrome, migraines, addictions, and other autoimmune diseases. Many of these same people are on medications and antibiotics, which influence the metabolism and aggravate the gluten reaction because the system becomes too acidic. It's getting more and more difficult to find anything apart from "Frankenfood" (genetically modified food; more about that in Chapter Five), and fast food when I want to dine out.

SUSTAINABLE FOOD? YOU BE THE JUDGE

In 2013, thirty-five percent, or one billion people worldwide, are obese, and 42 million children have a diet-related disease.

One out of eight children lacks access to proper nutrition, even though we have food over-production and crop production has grown thirty percent in twenty years.

Most of the crop production is focused on growing and selling corn, soy, and rice.

Grains are highly toxic due to genetic modification, pesticides, and herbicides.

People around the planet eat more meat than in the past, and the livestock industry is geared to feeding and raising animals for slaughter, which is costly and leaves much of the soil and water unsustainable.

From The Denver Museum of Natural History Food Show Exhibit. Summer, 2013

Difficult-to-digest foods can be very toxic for babies, celiacs, and older people. With age, food quality and flavor becomes a greater source of pleasure. For some older people, however, taste buds and sense of smell may fail, and there is greater craving for more salt, sugar, and spices to satisfy the palate. Many of these condiments in excess can lead to inflammation, increased immune deficiency, high cholesterol, high blood pressure, low thyroid or Hashimoto's disease, and other potentially fatal health challenges. Recently, I was diagnosed with a problem that many older women experience — an overactive bladder. My urologist says it is an allergic reaction to stimulants such as caffeine, chocolate, and spices. For a foodie, such as I am, it's been very hard to eliminate these tasty tidbits; however, I am seeing positive results. I counter sugar cravings by eating more butter and olive oil.

Despite this gluten challenge, I am healthier now than I have ever been, thanks to the gluten-free regime I follow closely. I am medication-free and fortify my system with specific Western and Chinese herbal supplements, which my trusted Chinese acupuncturist and naturopath prescribe. Whenever possible, I frequent local farmers' markets and health food supermarkets. Our local markets have begun to carry some organic and "gluten-free" foods. I choose to eat gluten-free, GMO and GE-free (genetically modified and genetically engineered), local, and organic. Gratefully, I enjoy more energy than ever before and also more depth of feeling and peace of mind.

If I do not follow my diet, I have mood swings, anxiety, joint aches, chapped lips, anxiety, insomnia, and fatigue. Fortunately, I know how to get back on track the next day. I use different tools along with diet: meditation, movement therapy, chakra work, breathing exercises, walks, journaling, and yoga.

I promise you that if you are consistent and committed to your gluten-free eating habits, you can improve on all levels almost immediately—sometimes in a matter of days. Opinions differ about a definite cure for gluten sensitivity, intolerance, and Celiac Disease. There are no definitive tests as yet—just indicators. (More about this in Chapter Two.) If you have not dealt with your gluten sensitivity for thirty years, it may take longer to get in balance and, you will have to follow the gluten-free trail for the rest of your life, with some flexibility as time goes on. You may become almost symptom-free in nine months if you hold to the dietary rules. Everyone should be tested for gliadin antibodies, especially for children aged three and under. The older you get the harder it is to heal from gluten-sensitivity or Celiac Disease.

As metabolism balances, many people lose or gain weight in the first month. You can also immediately experience less frequent migraines, fewer joint aches, digestive problems, and depression as you begin to detoxify. Doctors and nutritionists have learnewd more about gluten in the last few years. However, I suggest individualized discussion and research with a gluten expert, as each of us is unique. When we listen to our inner self and our body and feed our brain what it thrives on, we will find the path to the right diet and lifestyle. Then we can make this planet a healthier and happier place in which to live.

In Chapter Two, you will get some simple clarification about the gluten issue and suggestions about how to deal with it. I hope to demystify the subject and explain how you can incorporate an easy approach to your regime now, so that you will have a basic understanding of why a gluten-free diet is not healthy for everyone and can be dangerous for those who do not have gluten issues. I do advocate eating fewer grains or eliminating them completely, because they have been modified and are no longer authentic nutrition.

EAT REAL!

2

LIVING WITHOUT, FLOURISHING WITHIN

ILLUSTRATION BY JFS, AUTHOR

Sardines

One of my favorite foods is sardines. I feel secure when I eat them wild, fresh, or canned because they are so small they don't accumulate a large amount of mercury. This recipe is fun for breakfast, brunch, or a light supper. I eat them three times a week as recommended by James, my health practitioner, as they are so high in natural vitamin D. You can add minced and steamed kale to make it a complete meal.

FISHERMAN'S EGGS

SERVES 2

INGREDIENTS

125-gm can wild sardines
4 large, pastured, soy-free eggs
2 teaspoons organic Italian parsley leaves, finely chopped
3 organic scallions (green onions), minced
2 cloves organic garlic, minced

PREPARATION

Preheat oven to 375° F. and place an ovenproof dish inside while you assemble the ingredients.

Flake the sardines together with the parsley, garlic, and onion. Season generously with black pepper and tip into the heated ovenproof dish. Put in oven for five minutes.

Gently crack the eggs into a bowl.

Remove the sardines from the oven and carefully pour the eggs on top.

Season generously and return to oven for 15 minutes until the eggs are cooked but jiggly.

Let sit for a few minutes before serving so they congeal further.

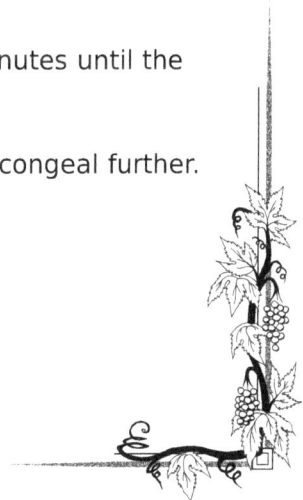

GLUTEN SENSITIVITY AND THE GLUTEN-FREE FAD

When I was sixty-eight years old, in 2004, my family doctor, diagnosed me as a possible Celiac. I had never heard of Celiac Disease or gluten before then, because it was a silent epidemic. The gluten issue already affected 1 in 300 people and many more were ignorant of this insidious issue. My doctor was a Celiac herself, and shared that it is very common with those of Jewish, Eastern European heritage. She advised me to omit all wheat from my diet. Around the same time, my naturopath diagnosed me with Sjogren's Disease, which is a similar, immune system inflammatory disease.

I also learned that CD and gluten sensitivity can also be contracted in traumatic circumstances such as extreme stress, surgical interventions, and childbirth. I had experienced all three. I also learned that women have celiac disease at a ratio of 3 to 1 when compared to men. I felt a shiver of fear when I put all these pieces of information together.

I began to research wheat allergies and food substitutes for wheat, rye, and barley, which were and still are what most nutritional experts tell people to avoid. After a few weeks of investigation and several experiments with eating diverse grains, I found the key to my continuous struggle for health. I was gluten intolerant to all grains!

Similar to 95% of Celiacs, for most of my life I had been unaware that I had this potentially life-threatening disease. I was simultaneously relieved to put a label on what might be wrong with my digestion and moods, and felt a shiver of fear that I might die. Did I have Celiac Disease? Would I, a chef who lived to eat delicious and unique foods on a daily basis and share feasts with my friends, have to deny myself my favorite foods?

By 2005, I was a food coach and cooking school director for Whole Foods Market — their first full time food coach at that time — a position I developed because many of my customers asked me for advice about what to eat when their doctor told them to eliminate wheat from their diet. At that time it took an average of 8 to 11 years and thousands of dollars (U.S. health insurance doesn't pay for celiac diagnosis or treatment) for a North American celiac to attempt a diagnosis.

I wanted to upgrade my diet to something beyond the Mediterranean Diet (vegetables and legumes with occasional red meat, other animal protein and lots of wheat and whole grains), which I had followed for more than 20 years when I lived in Tuscany. However, I had forgotten that from infancy I was allergic to wheat and other foods. When I fell in love with my Florentine husband to be (in the 1960s), I fell in love with Tuscan food, and together we devoured daily doses of pasta, bread, and pastries along with our protein and veggies. I was a glutton for gluten in those days, and I paid the price with depression, anxiety, nausea, and exhaustion.

Nutritionists and dieticians still promote the Mediterranean Diet as one of the world's healthiest nutritional regimes. However, beginning in the 1950s and up until the present time, most of America's produce in our supermarkets has been unlabeled, radiated and genetically modified (GMO). Nitrates and nitrite fertilizers are linked to increases in death rates from Alzheimer's, Parkinson's, and Diabetes. Italians have among the highest rate of Celiac Disease on the planet, because of all of the wheat products they consume in huge quantities. Italians crave their daily doses of wheat products to feel satisfied with their lives. The sugar from wheat and other grains acts like heroin on the brain and you become addicted in the same way you do with heroin, sugar, coffee and cigarettes. Today, the Italians are developing wheat-free wheat!

In comparison to the U.S., in Italy and other Western European countries, as well as India, Asia, and Africa, governmental food regulation law prohibits antibiotics, chemical fertilizers, or GMO. In 2013, Korea and Japan rejected any GMO products. As of March, 2013, Whole Foods Market became the very first supermarket to go completely GMO-Free. Whole Foods Market now has 3,300 Non-GMO Project–verified products, more than any other North American retailer. The trouble is that the packaging is usually toxic and not labeled accurately.

Until five years ago, I still didn't understand how deadly wheat was for me and continued to eat it occasionally. The latest research shows that the smallest amount of gluten can trigger inflammation and autoimmune reactions lasting for up to six months in gluten-sensitive individuals. Coffee has also been found to be one of the most harmful foods for those with gluten intolerance. It takes at least six months to recuperate from ⅛th-inch of gluten when you are gluten-intolerant or gluten-sensitive.

WHAT IS GLUTEN?

Gluten sensitivity is an autoimmune disease that occurs to some people when they eat gluten in any form. Wikipedia defines gluten as "…the composite of a gliadin and a glutenin, which is conjoined with starch in the endosperm of various grass-related grains. The prolamin and glutelin from wheat (gliadin, which is alcohol-soluble, and glutenin, which is only soluble in dilute acids or alkalis) constitute about 80% of the protein contained in wheat seed. Being insoluble in water, they can be purified by washing away the associated starch. Worldwide, gluten is a source of protein, both in foods prepared directly from sources containing it, and as an additive to foods otherwise low in protein." Gluten is a sticky protein that helps dough stick together. Bread is only 30,000 years old and was first made of cattails and ferns in Italy, Russia, and the Czechoslovakian republic.

A gluten or wheat allergy should not be confused with Celiac disease (CD). Celiac disease (also known as celiac sprue) affects the small intestine and is caused by an abnormal immune reaction to gluten. Usually diagnosed by a gastroenterologist, it is a digestive disease that can cause serious complications, including malnutrition, intestinal damage, and eventually fatal diseases such as cancer if left untreated. Gluten sensitivity itself is not a disease.

Research shows that as many as 40% of all Americans may be gluten sensitive, and 85% of Americans don't know they have this problem. Most of those affected are women. Soon the numbers will reach the billions worldwide if we include the fact that the whole planet has been affected by the U.S. food culture. More than one in one hundred have a severe form of this sensitivity that causes the autoimmune intestinal disease, CD, (Celiac Sprue).

Everyone should be screened for gluten sensitivity, which is associated with other life threatening diseases and can influence their growth. The root of all digestive diseases is due to autoimmune deficiency and inflammation caused by candida overgrowth, another symptom of gluten challenges. Although there are no definitive tests, science is getting closer to the answers.

The effects of gluten on the body and brain have similar consequences. When carbohydrates from grains, starchy vegetables, and most fruits convert to sugar, this creates The Metabolic Syndrome — uncontrollable cravings caused by lack of the neurotransmitter dopamine — that can become addictions and can alter the brain, body, and emotions. Celiac gypsies often crave bread and pastry, just as people who are alcoholics, drug addicts and smokers often develop wheat and sugar addictions, because they have a genetic disposition to the sugar in carbohydrates. Men crave sugar to repress their anxious feelings; women want sugar, especially chocolate, to quiet their stressful thoughts.

Sugar can also create an endless cycle of cravings and mood swings that lead to over-secretion of cortisol, a brain hormone that can lead to life-threatening diseases. Cortisol inhibits serotonin, the neurotransmitter that produces pleasurable feelings. I am happy to report that my cravings have diminished, partly due to the fact that my urologist has cured many women with over-active bladder with an allergy diet alone, and it's working for me. Check out this book on Kindle, only 99 cents: *The Krisiloff Anti-Inflammatory Diet* (Oct 15, 2010).

I find my most reliable way to check the gluten issue has always been to eliminate gluten and all grains, including those that are said to be "gluten-free," for ten days then put them back one at a time and test your reaction. I always feel more emotional, irritable or have a stomach ache after I have even the smallest amount of gluten. Once this gluten-free fad begins to slow down, the truth will be out— No grains are gluten-free because they are carbohydrates that convert to sugar. The sugar causes more inflammation and results in immune disease. The multi-billion dollar, gluten-free industry that has flourished in the last few years will crash, and this very dangerous fad will go down the drain with the false gluten-free products. Better still, the people with major digestive problems will get the truth from gluten experts instead of corporations who make a living from the lie about gluten-free products. I want to encourage people to slow down when they grocery shop, read label details, and call the manufacturer with any doubts.

ALLERGY vs. INTOLERANCE AND SENSITIVITY

Gluten-sensitivity is an autoimmune disease that causes inflammation of the lower intestines. All nutrients we consume are transported in the bloodstream to be absorbed by our small intestines. If the villi—which are tiny, finger-like projections in the small intestines—lay flattened because of wheat and gluten sensitivities they are no longer able to absorb nutrients. We then risk anemia and other life threatening diseases such as cancer, arthritis, and neurological imbalances such as depression, mood swings, autism, and ADHD. There are over 250 possible symptoms related to gluten problems, which has made it very difficult to diagnose in the past. Gluten issues also limit our ability to digest vitamin supplements. I took supplements for years and never noticed any major benefits. I was also anemic.

Gluten intolerance is often inherited. It can also be caused by trauma, such as surgery and pregnancy. Scott Adams. an MD, celiac and founder of the websites *www.celiac.com* and *www.glutenfreemall.com*, has posted in his blog research published in 1995 by Luigi Greco of the University of Naples concluding that gluten intolerance "is strongly linked to specific genetic markers which have indeed required thousands of years to develop and be selected: the 'population genetic' time is of this dimension, while the changes in the environment and in the food we eat, requiring centuries."

This pediatric study also notes that "in the suburbs of Naples, only 25 years ago, infectious diarrhea was the main killer (25% on an infant mortality rate of 100 per thousands live births). The vast majority of gluten intolerance occurred among these poor infants."

In 2010, the Italians had the highest rate of wheat and gluten intolerance in the world. They are also better informed than Americans about CD. The Irish and Middle Eastern people are also high on the list for gluten problems. Yet, not all populations of the world were exposed to the gluten protein molecule, gliadin, in wheat, rye, and barley. "The vast majority of mankind, after the development of agriculture, lived on maize, rice, sorghum, millet, and tubers: all gluten-free. All of [these cultures] did not undergo the selective pressure of gluten intolerance."

The beginning of farming, and the use of irrigation, allowed the survival, and expansion, of polyploid (an organism with more than two sets of chromosomes) grains. Wild wheat first appeared around 6000 years B.C. when the genetic uniformity caused a considerable rise in stability and yield for wheat. In 10,000 B.C., the early farmer was induced to begin a program of a progressive and rapid replacement of the wild species of edible plants. Genetic variability of grains was essential in order to adapt the plant to the very different environmental conditions of different areas. But the yield was generally low, and 12,000 years ago it was difficult to pick these grains, hence the Neolithics attempted to select varieties which could retain the seed longer in order to allow for a harvest.

HSP LIFEGUIDE

Be careful to eat only wild fish and check the mercury content at:
http://cantonbecker.com/wp-content/uploads/2012/04/mercury-fish-seafood-chart.pdf

SAFEST SEAFOOD

Contaminated with the least mercury:

Anchovies
Butterfish
Catfish
Clam
Crab (Domestic)
Crawfish/Crayfish
Croaker (Atlantic)
Flounder
Haddock (Atlantic)
Hake
Herring
Mackerel
(N. Atlantic, Chub)
Mullet
Oyster
Perch (Ocean)
Plaice
Pollock
Salmon
(Wild, Canned or Fresh)
Farmed Salmon
(might contain PCBs)
Sardine
Scallop
Shad (American)
Shrimp
Sole (Pacific)
Squid (Calamari)
Tilapia
Trout (Freshwater)
Whitefish
Whiting

FORMALDEHYDE DETECTED IN SUPERMARKET FISH IMPORTED FROM ASIA

"A large number of fish imported from China and Vietnam and sold in at least some U.S. supermarkets contain unnatural levels of formaldehyde, a known carcinogen, according to tests performed and verified by researchers at a North Carolina chemical engineering firm and North Carolina State University."

The team tested whether or not levels of formaldehyde increased in cuts of fish as they aged, but the levels remained the same. They also tested the same species harvested from both Chinese and U.S. companies, finding that the Chinese-caught fish contained formaldehyde, while the U.S.-caught fish of the same species did not.

According to the National Oceanic and Atmospheric Association, the U.S. imports approximately 91% of its seafood. China alone accounts for approximately 89% of global aquaculture production. Appealing Products' formaldehyde test costs approximately $1 per swab, which is applied to a cut of fish and turns purple in the presence of formaldehyde. The company has shipped 100,000 tests to Bangladesh and anticipates orders from companies in other Asian countries. More information on the tests can be found at *formaldehydetests.com*.

Documented instances of intentional formaldehyde contamination of food have occurred in China, Vietnam, Indonesia and Thailand.

Source:
http://www.foodsafetynews.com/2013/09/formaldehyde-detected-in -supermarket-fish-imported-fr om-asia/#.UjbWINIy0rU

http://wakeupcallnews.blogspot.com.au/2013/09 /formaldehyde-detected-in-supermarket.html

The focus on gluten seems based on simple economics. "In our part of the world grains had for centuries been selected in order to improve their homogeneity and productivity, but soon (Roman times or before?), another desirable quality was preferred: the ability to stick, to glue up a dough to improve bread making. Early bread-making activities pushed towards grains that contained greater amounts of a structural protein, which greatly facilitated the bread making: the gluten."

Gluten was not chosen because of its nutritional value (it is a protein with relatively low nutritional value) but for its commercial qualities. Over the last 200 years of our modern age, active genetic selection and genetic modification have changed the aspect of the original wheat from few grains and little gluten, to huge wheat production with added gluten (50% of the protein content), and chemical additives to preserve the shelf life.

We no longer eat the original wheat grain, and we are still too young as human beings to digest the adulterated wheat we can buy in today's markets and bakeries. No one does well when they eat wheat, but many people are more sensitive to grains than others. Our intolerance and sensitivity can also begin or increase as we age.

Adams' post, however, suggests that the majority of mankind never lived on bread alone.

CROSS-GRAINS

Not all "wheat- and gluten-free" labels are to be trusted, as some of these grains, such as millet and oat, are often grown near gluten-carrier grains, or are processed in the same location as wheat and soy, which are usually GMO. Another cause of wheat and gluten sensitivity is too much grain consumption. Even an excess of "Gluten-Free" goodies can lead to carbohydrate overload, a precursor of some emotional disorders such as schizophrenia, depression, or diabetes due to the high amount of sugar. Sugar is not metabolized well by the pancreas. High sugar content, fructose, and starchy carbohydrates lead to excessive insulin release, which can lead to falling blood sugar levels, or hypoglycemia. Hypoglycemia, in turn, causes the brain to secrete glutamate in levels that can cause agitation, depression, anger, anxiety, panic attacks, and an increase in suicide risk.

A PERSONALIZED DIET

I was born with an allergy to cow's milk and most dairy products due to the casein and was raised on goat milk. Many people don't digest dairy well. Cows are fed corn and soy, which are usually high in GMO. Even grass fed cattle is often "finished" with grains. I only eat soy-free eggs, and I try to find those that come from chickens who are pasture-fed and not fed corn or other grains. I eat nuts and Granny Smith apples. Lately, I don't miss many of my favorite foods of the past or sugar. For the most part, I crave protein and healthy animal and vegetable fat.

When I treat myself to an occasional grass-fed rib-eye steak or clod-cut of buffalo, I am as completely satisfied as any other carnivore. I do check, however, that the grass-fed beef or buffalo wasn't finished with grains before slaughter.

I experiment with my Gluten-Free regime, diligently read labels and continue to research what to eat and test my results, in order to share my findings through lectures, consultations and writing. I find the more I learn and the closer I follow my personalized gluten-free lifestyle, the more energy and disease resistance I experience. The biggest secret that makes my life much easier is to keep it simple. I eat protein and veggies for breakfast, lunch and dinner. Dessert is a poached Granny Smith apple or frozen organic raspberries, soaked and air-dried raw walnuts and pumpkin seeds with a quality salt. Even though I regret that I was in denial about this sensitivity for so many years, I am grateful beyond words that I am able to research and adventure with this lifestyle now, and that I have found a dependable path towards my well-being that I can share with others.

As I was getting ready to publish this book, I ran across a newsletter post from a major supplement retailer that sells "natural" supplements and food. I was not surprised to see that their "gluten-free" snacks contain grains and sugar.

Gluten-Free — The Fascinating New Food Phenomenon
Welcome to Gluten-Free 101

You've heard all this talk about Gluten-Free diets… Fad? Folly? Food for thought? What's the story about a gluten-free diet? We're here to separate the wheat from the chaff… or maybe just separate you from wheat. Or not.

Talk about buzz! Gluten's got it. Ranging from nutritional-purist-true-believers, aka "Sustainable Wellness Evangelists," to concerned mothers worried about their child's food allergies, to determining school lunch programs, to TV news shows looking for the latest bad-news story, the topic seems everywhere. You see "We Have Gluten-Free" promos at convenience stores!

There's this from The Wheat Foods Counsel:

> **A new survey from market research firm the NPD Group finds that America is cutting gluten out of its diet in a big way. Just under one-third of 1,000 respondents agreed with the statement: "I'm trying to cut back/avoid Gluten in my diet."**

That's the highest level since the company added gluten consumption to the surveys it does about Americans' eating habits in 2009. *Time* labeled the gluten-free movement #2 on its top-10 list of food trends for 2012.

As food fads go, though, this one's not only enormous, it's enormously expensive—and many of us paying a premium to avoid gluten are doing so without any legitimate medical reason.

Is this about gluten or bread, i.e., money?

http://www.puritan.com/newsletter/20130816/gluten?scid=27357&cmp=yml-_-20130816-_-gluten

Many of these new "gluten-free" products contain GMO, sugar, fructose, chemical additives, cross-grains, cross contaminants, and more. Children, older people, and pregnant women are more affected by these foods than the average person.

Evidence suggests the G-F diet has become a dangerous fad. I am more concerned than ever that people are embracing it for the wrong reasons: to lose weight, because it is the latest thing, or because they hope to cure their digestive problems. People need to find out if they are actually gluten challenged; otherwise, they can become anemic or develop other diseases without a diagnosis.

There is not a 100% definitive test on the market as yet. Dr. Peter Osborne's 3-step cellular antibody test comes closest, but there are still false positives and false negatives. As I continue to experiment with my gluten-free regime, I continue to research what I eat, test my results by how I feel, and read labels so I can share my findings through lectures, consultations, and writing. The more I learn, and the closer I follow my personalized gluten-free lifestyle, the more energy and disease resistance I experience. Across-the-board diets don't work.

I am grateful beyond words that I am able to research and adventure with this lifestyle, and that I have found a dependable path towards my well-being. I love to research the growing variety of gluten-free online recipes and discover new cookbooks to enhance my gluten-free repertoire. I've even improved my baking skills!

I encourage you to get over any sense of intimidation, boredom or distaste about the true gluten-free regime. Achieve better health for yourself and your family and friends!

3

DIET VS. REGIME

Primo Piatto (First Course)
Sugo al Pomodoro

Mama Bianca was my beautiful Florentine mother-in-law. Bianca learned to cook from her Uncle Tebaldo, who was a chef in the fine hotels of Florence during the turn of the 18th century. She was a perfectionist and didn't let me do anything in the kitchen but watch her for the first six months that I lived in her home as her daughter-in-law. After that, I was able to do some chopping and slicing. When I separated from my husband and left Italy, my friends in Denver told me what a good cook I was. I was surprised that I had learned everything I needed to begin a new career.

Mama Bianca's Classic Tuscan Tomato Sauce

SERVES 4

INGREDIENTS

3 Tbsp. grapeseed oil

4 cloves garlic, chopped

1 can organic, whole San Marzano tomatoes or fresh, ripe, chopped cherry tomatoes

½ cup Italian parsley, chopped

½ cup fresh basil leaves, torn, or 1 Tbsp. dried and powdered

1 Tbsp. olive oil

PREPARATION

Sauté the garlic in the grapeseed oil until light gold. Be careful not to burn or you will have to start over.

Add the tomatoes and simmer for 10 minutes, or until sauce is thickened

Add olive oil and sprinkle with basil and parsley.

Sprinkle with Parmesan, Asiago, or Romano if desired

Pour over protein or veggies and serve warm or room temperature

Chef's Note

This makes an excellent base for poached eggs and can be an entire meal at any time of the day. Great for unexpected guests, as it only takes a few minutes to make if you have some frozen sauce in the freezer.

Puree this sauce for a different texture, and one that is better for smaller vegetables. This sauce is great with raw or grilled cherry tomatoes.

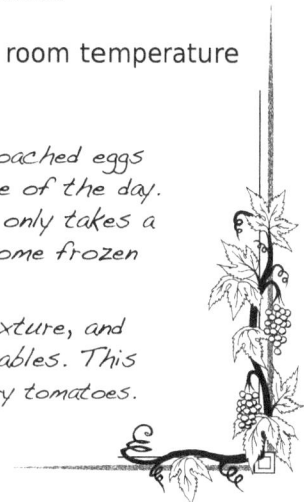

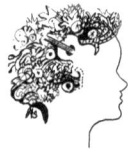

> *Try the alternative pasta with this that is made from bean threads and is grain-free!*
>
> *This is also wonderful to use with most vegetables, such as kale and green beans. To add protein, use pastured chicken, turkey, grass-fed ground bison or beef.*

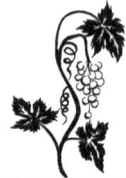

*A*s an eight-year-old Jewish Princess about to bloom, I was a young rebel who yearned to be as free as a gypsy. I was dealing with a sour tummy and acid disposition as well as many food allergies. I had eczema and was chronically depressed. I waited each day for my prince in shining armor (and amour) to appear on his white stallion and carry me off to Paris. Even though our noveau rich and sometimes poor family (due to my father's business risks) was not religious, they rigidly conformed to the social mores of the fifties. I knew there was something better than Denver and being polite. Later, as an 11-year old, I fell in virtual love with a famous actor of that time and continued to immerse myself in art books and French novels. I dreamed of being an artist and studying art in Paris. I thought I would marry a Frenchman and love happily ever after.

Now I am a Theosophist, a marketing coach for creative entrepreneurs, and no longer a princess. The school of hard knocks has shown me how to develop my individual eating style and essence. I have always journaled about my life, and a few years ago I was compelled to write this G-F memoir cookbook, because the gluten-free fad is dangerous. Baby Boomers, my age group and audience, are free-form eaters as a whole. They are impulsive with their food choices and often overweight, as I have been. After years of avoiding a healthy diet regime, they have shocked their metabolism by inconsistent diets, and are beginning to experience bad digestion, as well as anonymous aches and pains. They are often confused about what foods they should eat to feel good.

We are all unique, and no single diet is good for everyone, but I have found a regime that works for me and my clients and friends. I dislike the word diet. I prefer the French *regime*, or the English *regimen*. Most Europeans view their personal as an integral part of their individualized lifestyle, with adventure, family, laughter, love, and legacy as essential ingredients that add flavor to their daily lives. They are not obsessed with issues of weight, as many Americans are, and enjoy their food without guilt or deprivation. Some overeat and suffer from gout, but on the whole, the Mediterranean Diet suits them well.

My culinary adventure travels began when I was a naïve and *almost* virginal age eighteen. I had crossed the Atlantic Ocean on a Dutch ship to study art and French in Paris — my childhood dream. I threw myself into the throes of a passionate attraction to a dashing and handsome Florentine man whom I met in Florence. His name was Massimo, and he brought me succulent grapes to eat after we made love in little pension rooms in Florence. I met him on the romantic Ponte Vecchio Bridge where Dante first met Beatrice in 1283. She inspired him to revolutionize the Italian language. I wanted to inspire Massimo.

I was on a side trip from art school in Paris. He guessed my name and told me he had dated my best friend one year previous to our meeting. I knew he was the soul mate I had searched for since I was a child.

I immediately redesigned myself as an American version of a typical Florentine young woman. I supplied him with his daily dose of affection, sex and pasta in Paris, London, New York, San Francisco, and throughout all of our other travels — even when I had to cook the pasta in a teapot. In the midst of my passion, I forgot I was allergic to wheat and other foods! I didn't think about my allergy, in spite of occasional tummy problems, headaches, and intense mood swings.

I had never met anyone who had been to Italy and had never been to an authentic Italian restaurant before I went to Italy at age eighteen. He was my Dante and led me through the many levels of Italian mythology and cultural traditions. He also introduced me to the marvels of Tuscan food as we wandered the streets of Florence and nibbled tasty morsels from carts, delis, and *trattoria* along the way.

Apart from the wheat, the Mediterranean Diet is very close to the Paleo Diet, which is beginning to be popular at this time. It is a diet that is based on animal protein and no grains, very different from what the USDA recommends today and similar to the diet we ate as Neanderthals. This is a diet that has replaced the gluten-free diet as a fad because many consumers who had a gluten problem found they felt sick when they ate grains.

After I had a brief affair with Massimo, I returned to Paris, where I studied art and French. After a few months, Massimo followed me, and we lived together in Paris and London. My mother was worried because she had no sign that I would ever return to Denver, so my meager allowance of $150 a month stopped. I returned to my parents in Denver and then on to San Francisco to finish my art degree. Massimo followed me there, where he modeled in my school, The California School of Fine Arts.

When I graduated, his visa expired, and he returned to Florence. I was working in my first job as an editorial assistant at Putnam publishing and then found a fascinating job in an elite art gallery on Madison Avenue. I still had a dream of becoming a famous artist and living in Paris. One day, Massimo surprised me in the gallery after I had written him I had a boyfriend, and we began to live together again. Before I met Bianca, my future mother-in-law, Massimo was my impatient and critical cooking teacher. There were many cooking adventures, amidst my tears, and his shouts. He returned to Florence again when his visa ran out, and I went home to Denver for a year.

After a year of tearful longing and frustration at my parents' home in Denver for Massimo's letters, which were practically non-existent, I wrote Massimo an ultimatum that he had to come to Denver and take me away (my childhood prince charming fantasy?). One day, I received a phone call that Massimo was in jail for smuggling gold into the U.S. on one of his trips to New York. While he was in Florence, he had also been selling leather goods to women he had met in his shop when he went to NYC, and also made them an Italian meal in their apartments at private trunk showings. My father set bail through one of his connections, and Massimo came to Denver to meet my parents and my brother Douglas for the first time.

My mother had enough of my moping about Massimo. I just wanted to live with him, not marry. But that wasn't what my mother wanted. She persuaded my father to do a sales job on Massimo so he would promise to marry me. It worked and we had a rushed marriage in my Denver home, as he was still on bail and had to return to New York for his trial. He was on a scholarship at the Actor's Studio at the time. That's another story. After our Italian/Jewish judge married us, we had brunch in the finest hotel in Denver, where my parents had had their own wedding brunch. My Denver friend Maria, who was a Florentine, was maid of honor, and threw up during multiple trips to the bathroom during our elegant brunch. She told me a few years later that she knew Massimo's reputation and didn't want to tell me because I was so much in love with him.

After a brief honeymoon in San Francisco, we flew back to Manhattan for the smugglng trial. Massimo's New Yorker lawyer, an actor friend from the Actor's Studio, never showed at the trial due to a heart attack, and as Massimo had no legal representation, he was deported. The gold was confiscated, and he had to leave immediately. After a couple of months, I packed up our belongings and quit my job in the art gallery. I returned to Florence to live with my mother-in-law, Bianca, for six months. In the next few years, we moved to various romantic rentals in the Tuscan hill towns, an ancient villa outside Florence, and then a carriage house in the hills directly above Florence.

When we lived with Bianca, my Zen-style, culinary *maestra*, she let me watch her, but she wouldn't let me touch the food. It was like the Zen of cooking lessons because she made me watch, and my desire to emulate her and cook grew at each meal preparation. We had two four-course meals a day in her ancient, tiny fifth-floor walkup across from the Duomo in the center of Florence. She had been tutored in Tuscan cuisine by her Tuscan Uncle Corrado, a chef in the fine hotels of Florence at the turn of the 18th Century. Bianca was an amazing cook who sang operatic arias as she cooked, and I learned all her classic, authentic Tuscan culinary secrets. Our small family ate, laughed, and drank local Chianti wine as I learned Traditional Tuscan cooking through osmosis. When I opened her kitchen shutters, the window was filled by the Duomo cupola. It was so hot at lunchtime that the perspiration rolled down our faces as we enjoyed our *spaghetti con vonghole*.

I became pregnant in 1966 with our son, Sacha, and our gypsy life continued as we moved from Florence to a one-room apartment in Rome so that Massimo could pursue his career as an actor, even though we both preferred Florence. I was thrilled to receive a scholarship to the Calclografia Nazionale, an Italian institution from the 1500s that reprints ancient and modern graphics by hand. Massimo pursued his career as an actor and landed his first part in a film as a

Persian soldier in John Houston's blockbuster film, *The Bible*. We both missed Florence and preferred it to Rome and spent as much time as possible in Florence when Massimo wasn't working as an actor.

I had not yet heard of gluten-intolerance or *Celiac Disease*. I was nauseous from my pregnancy and at the same time didn't understand why I became more and more toxic and extremely ill with stomach aches, headaches, depression, and extreme irritability. I was miserable. I was still ignoring my wheat allergy and fighting with Massimo over my attempts to please him with my cooking. We continued to eat the normal Italian diet based on wheat in the form of pasta and twice-daily, fresh-baked wheat rolls.

In December of 1966, the year of the devastating flood in Florence, we had a healthy son, Sacha. I nursed him and continued to eat pasta and bread — still in denial about the connection between wheat and my mood swings and nausea. When Sacha began to eat solids, I gave him cream of wheat (*semolina*) with his liver and veggies — I didn't consider the fact that he might have inherited my allergies. I hadn't learned yet about gluten, and he had no visible sign of any dietary problems. He is now gluten-sensitive.

I still was worried about my own diet, mood swings, and nausea. Sacha, on the other hand, was always a voracious eater as an infant and had no sign of allergies. He gobbled up everything on his plate, even throughout the verbal and emotional battles Massimo and I had about my cooking.

Sacha is now 47 years old; at age 40 he discovered that he did inherit the gluten intolerance gene. I was miserable. It is paradoxical that Italian was never my favorite cuisine. My main culinary efforts were to please my food-fussy Florentine husband.

At the American Express office in Rome one day, I was lucky enough to meet an American *shiatsu* teacher from the East-West Macrobiotic Center in Boston. Serendipity or answered prayers? His treatments and a rice-based diet help me immediately, and I become a core member of the Rome Macrobiotic Center. His partner was a sophisticated older man and macrobiotic from Genoa, Italy. I became a macrobiotic chef and kitchen manager in their tiny, chic apartment in the center of Rome that catered macro feasts to international actors and the aging Italian aristocracy who wanted longevity. I felt much better when I followed this extreme diet for a few years. The *shiatsu* treatments and a rice-based diet helped me immediately but made the dining situation at home with Massimo much worse.

At that time, there was a lot of controversy about macrobiotics, which the hippies had adopted. Some thought it could be life-threatening, and rightly so, as it was a complicated lifestyle, and not just a diet. Few followed it as with as much rigor as I did. I actually took my food to restaurants and dinner parties, despite my friends mocking taunts for being too much an "Americana." Our restaurant finally collapsed when the two owners had a very yang fight and tore the phone out of the wall in front of my shocked eyes. (Too much yang and not enough yin balance.) At this point, I didn't know where to turn. I was fed up with Massimo's demands and possessiveness. I was sick and knew I had to heal, if only for Sacha. I was his only security, and I was falling apart.

In the late 1960s and early 1970s in Rome, I was still a wife and mother, but spent less and less time with Massimo. He went out with his friends every night after dinner to "look for acting jobs and network," and I stayed home with Sacha. Then, one of our macrobiotic restaurant clients offered me a position as kitchen manager for a macrobiotic restaurant she was opening, so I went for lessons to become a certified chef and kitchen manager. I also became a pioneer American Radical Feminist who organized demonstrations with the leading international feminists of the time in Piazza Navona.

At the same time, I became a very successful fashion designer that sold high-end wearable art to fashion models and actresses in a boutique at the bottom of the Spanish Steps in Rome. I found someone to make the patterns and sew the basic designs and was thrilled that the boutique manager bought everything I made. My designs were very popular and had a definite Gypsy-Hippie flair.

In the autumn of 1974, my father phoned me in Rome in the middle of the night to tell me to return to Denver immediately. My mother, Sarabelle, was dying from breast cancer. I left the next day and returned to Denver to care for her. I left Sacha with Massimo and moved into my parents' tiny apartment, and slept on the couch. My mother lived for six months longer than the doctors predicted because I cooked all her meals in the macrobiotic tradition. She died in my arms in the hospital. I rented a two-bedroom apartment next door to the Denver Botanic Gardens, the same area as where I grew up, and began my first therapy sessions. I soon became part of a group of radical feminists who were studying to become therapists.

Three months later, Sacha flew alone at seven years old to join me in Denver. I enrolled him in a private grammar school where I taught French and Art to help pay for part of his tuition. My father crumbled when he lost his business due to the financial crash in the 1980s, and was severely depressed due to my mother's death. So he came to live with Sacha and me for six months. After a year, when my father went back to his apartment, my brother, Doug, divorced and also came to live with me for a few months. I had no idea what my own divorce would mean to Sacha or me, and I didn't want to think about it. I tried to maintain a cheery front in spite of my severe depression, and I acquired our darling English Sheep-German Shepherd puppy, Frisbee, who lived with us as a loyal friend and babysitter until Sacha graduated from college.

After a few years at the private elementary school, Sacha transferred to a public junior high school and the public high school in Denver (where my father and I were past students). Over those difficult years as a single mother, Massimo would surprise us with occasional visits from Italy. Once he came galloping down our street dressed in a bikini with a papier-mache horse head on his head.

In high school, Sacha's school had no computers, and I didn't want him to start college without those skills. I enrolled in a computer class so I could teach an introductory computer familiarization class for the PTA and Sacha's teachers. We organized a fundraiser, and Apple and IBM donated computers. We built the high school's first computer lab, with the help of Denver's leading architect who donated his services, and donations from the parents. The lab won a prize for the best computer lab in Colorado high schools. I was relieved that Sacha would go to college with some computer knowledge. However, at home, Sacha's rebellions were too obvious to ignore, and my temper grew shorter despite our family therapy.

I didn't know I was gluten-sensitive, and I had no idea that Sacha might have inherited this insidious disease. I know now that my father had all the signs and symptoms of gluten sensitivity or intolerance because he had eczema; however, we continued to eat pasta and bread.

4

SYMPTOMS AND DEFINITIONS

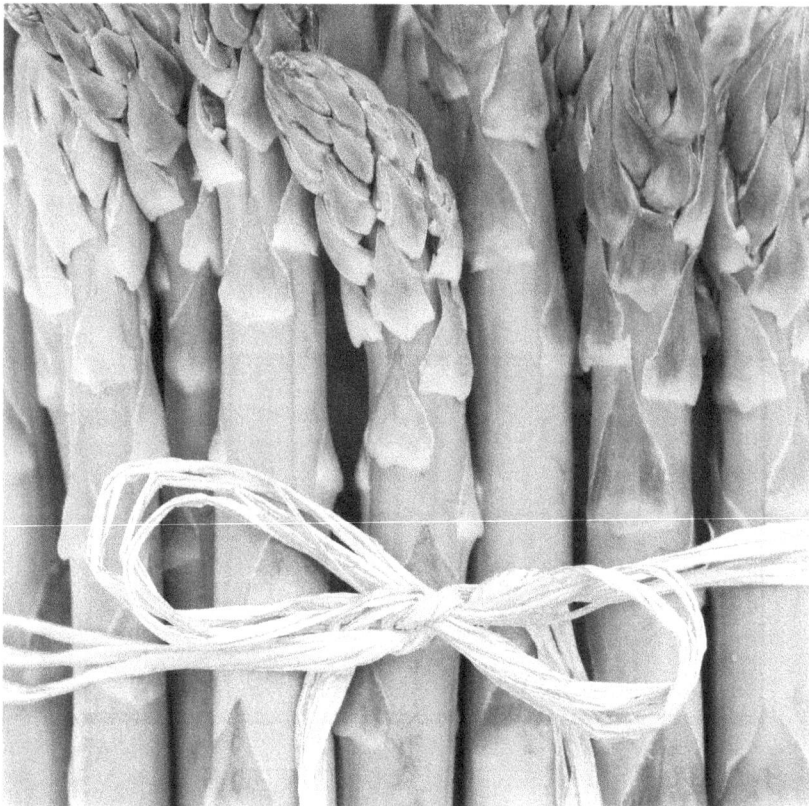

Contorno
(SIDE DISH)

Zia (Auntie) Norena was Massimo's aunt, Zio Tebaldo's wife, and a fabulous cook. They lived in Abetone, Tuscany, at the foot of the Dolomites with their family. All their vegetables, fruit, and livestock were organic and sustainable. Whenever Massimo and I visited, Tebaldo would take us to forage for Porcini mushrooms before sunrise. Norena would cook up the Porcini mushrooms we found in a sauce with a hare Tebaldo had caught. She would make polenta with the sauce. It was one of the best dishes I ever tasted. She would serve it with her asparagus as a side dish or antipasto. Use this cooked asparagus for delicious risotto, pasta, or soup.

ZIA NORENA'S ASPARAGUS: BETTER THAN BROCCOLI

SERVES 2

INGREDIENTS

1 bunch of fresh, organic asparagus
2 Tbsp Organic olive oil
3 Tbsp. organic Parmesan cheese grated
1 teaspoon lemon zest — freshly grated lemon rind
Himalayan salt
Lemon pepper to taste

PREPARATION

Snap the asparagus stalks off where they bend.

Steam the asparagus for 2 minutes, or until bright green and crunchy.

Remove the asparagus to a bowl while still hot; toss them in a bowl with the olive oil, Parmesan, and lemon rind.

Salt and pepper to taste.

Serve warm or at room temperature as an antipasto or side dish.

Wrap the stalks with prosciutto for a special treat.

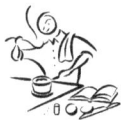

Chef's Note

Grill or roast the asparagus after marinating in salt, lemon pepper, and olive oil. Wrap with thin slices of prosciutto when cooked. Poached asparagus and chicken broth pureed makes a delicious cold soup. Add some fresh tarragon or basil.

GLUTEN-FREE DIET FAD MYTHS

Have you ever experienced the following problem? A few hours after a pleasant meal, you start getting what may be a gluten reaction, (glutening). Your symptoms show up as digestive pain, anxiety, and/or skin problems, because you have been exposed to hidden gluten in the food or environment. It often takes only a tiny bit of gluten to become glutened and experience a reaction. For some who are gluten sensitive or intolerant, these symptoms can take up to several weeks to disappear.

Researchers are discovering more and more about gluten-related foods and health issues. However, the media hasn't picked up or shared the most recent specifics of the scientific, documented research with its readers and is still promoting the gluten-free fad I am frustrated about this because my own research for this book tells me that the larger percentage of gluten-free products on the shelf in health food stores and supermarkets is not gluten-free. These corporate-sponsored products contain cross-grains and will contribute to the growth of gluten in the digestive tract of millions of unsuspecting people who have joined the gluten-free fad. The 2014 FDA labeling regulation for gluten is too high and not specific enough. If a consumer is gluten-sensitive or intolerant, has CD, or hasn't investigated the gluten challenge, or read the labels carefully, and called the manufacturer when unsure of the content, the problem is not resolved. Glutening often leads to immune system inflammation and major diseases such as cancer, rheumatoid arthritis, heart disease, macular degeneration, and neurological and brain diseases such as schizophrenia and ADD.

In an article titled "Scientists Have Discovered That Celiac Disease Can Be the Root Cause for Most Neurological Disorders" on *Sott.com*,[1] Caryn Talty, of the *Healthy-Family.org*, quotes K. Mustalahti, of the Pediatric Research Centre, University of Tampere, Finland:

> "K. Mustalahti, of the Pediatric Research Centre, University of Tampere, Finland states: 'Recently, a growing body of distinct neurologic conditions has been connected to untreated celiac disease, mainly in middle aged adults. These manifestations are usually chronic, such as occipital lobe epilepsy with cerebral calcifications, cerebellar ataxia, progressive leukoencephalopathy, and dementia. Seven-percent of all untreated celiac disease patients are diagnosed on the basis of various neurological symptoms. Although earlier studies reported neurologic

disorders in patients with classical gluten enteropathy, some recent studies report neurologic symptoms in otherwise asymptomatic celiac disease patients. The pathogenic mechanisms underlying neurological disorders remain obscure, but immunological mechanisms are implicated. In few cases neurological symptoms seem to be alleviated by gluten-free diet but mostly the disorders are permanent. [...] The current criteria for celiac disease may give the false impression that celiac disease is purely a gastrointestinal disorder with manifest small-bowel mucosal lesion.'"

Excerpts cited from: "Unusual Manifestations of Celiac Disease,"
Indian Journal of Pediatrics, Volume 73, August 2006.

I am a researcher, not a doctor or nutritionist, and do not claim to have answers to anyone's health problems apart from my own. I know that in 2007 my symptoms of mood swings, low energy, eczema, anxiety, psoriasis, nausea, and more began to disappear the first week I began my gluten-free diet. I lost 30 pounds in four months as I ate everything I wanted to without the gluten, and another 10 pounds a year later without dieting.

The gluten-free diet wasn't a fad when I began. Most people and doctors were not familiar with the definition of gluten, much less the dangers, even though it had sometimes been mentioned in medical schools since the 1940s. Much progress has been made in the last five or six years as regards available research. People, however, still often see several different specialists and spend months or years of illness, and spend thousands of dollars to finally identify gluten as the cause of their health problems. In most cases, the gluten issue is not covered by health insurance.

As I look back to my twenty years in Tuscany, I muse about how different my life, as a wife and mother in another culture, would have been if I had been gluten-free since childhood. Even though I was a Highly Sensitive Person, I believe there would have been less irritability and emotionalism on my part and less volatile arguments about small matters with my mother, husband Massimo, and my son Sacha. I would have had much less anxiety and worry about how I was raising my son and more relaxing and enjoyable times with my family and friends. I would have made sure that Massimo and Sacha were gluten-free, as well, and thus provided a healthier base for our family core.

I am happy to share that today my son, Sacha, my three-year-old granddaughter, Bianca, and her mother are now mostly gluten-free and very careful about the rest of their diets. After seven years on a mainly G-F diet, I feel like a new, 77-years-young woman on this regime.

About one-third of the world population carries the genetic background for gluten intolerance — but only one percent of people have it. Before gluten causes can be tested in the lab, researchers must develop an animal model with celiac disease or do an intestinal biopsy. Italy, Ireland, the U.S., and the Middle East have the highest incidence of gluten challenges because they eat so much wheat and other carbohydrates such as potatoes and beans. All carbohydrates convert to sugar and trigger the metabolic syndrome in those who are gluten-challenged.

Today's gluten-free fad is very detrimental to everyone who doesn't understand the specifics of their personal digestive or emotional challenges, especially those that are gluten-sensitive and have no symptoms. Many people also will go on and off the diet to lose weight or just out of curiosity. Gluten is not something to be toyed with.

In 2012, new information led to the proof that all grains can be connected with gluten challenges, even though there may be no visible proof of connection to actual gluten. A person can be sensitive to a cross-grain, such as rice, millet, oats, soy or corn, because they consume beef or chicken that was fed GMO, antibiotics, pesticides or hormones. They can have a similar reaction as to CD. It's a complicated problem. Even though they do not contain the gluten protein, cross-grains contribute to inflammation of the immune system due to the carbohydrates that convert to sugar. Quinoa is a seed and not a grain, but is often processed with wheat and is considered a cross-grain because it mimics grains when it is digested and metabolized.

HOW DO GLUTEN SENSITIVITY, GLUTEN INTOLERANCE, AND CELIAC DISEASE DIFFER?

Dr. Daniel DiGiacomo, MD, MPH, is board certified in Gastroenterology and a research assistant at Columbia University in New York. He confirmed in data presented in Las Vegas at the October 24, 2012 American College of Gastroenterology Annual Scientific Meeting that the incidence of non-celiac gluten sensitivity (NCGS) is about half that of celiac disease.

"A growing number of patients are being found to have non-celiac gluten sensitivity," Dr. DiGiacomo told *Healio.com* and other audience participants in a recent lecture. "Unfortunately, there is not much clinical data, nor published studies, on non-celiac gluten sensitivity. We thought this would be the perfect opportunity to take an epidemiological approach and study non-celiac gluten sensitivity, on a national level."

Researchers evaluated data from the Continuous National Health and Nutrition Survey between 2009 and 2010, which included 7,762 participants aged six years and older. The report says that the prevalence of NCGS, defined as undertaking a gluten-free diet following the exclusion of celiac disease, was determined within this cohort, along with demographics and health status for those with the condition. Forty-nine participants were diagnosed with NCGS. This difference was closer to significance among patients aged 65 years or older.

"Our study, albeit preliminary in its nature, depicts non-celiac gluten sensitivity as a disorder that is less common than celiac disease," DiGiacomo said, adding that the results are preliminary due to sample size. "This is in contrast to prior expectations, that gluten sensitivity is several times more common than celiac disease. Overall, caution should be used, whether it is in the home or the doctor's office, when deciding to partake in the gluten-free diet. Unless one is afflicted with a gluten-related disorder, this diet is most likely unnecessary, and may present with some potential long-term health risks if not followed properly."

Celiac disease, an immune reaction to eating the protein gluten, is far more than an occasional tummy upset. Mayo Clinic research suggests the disease is becoming a major public health issue. Although the cause is unknown, celiac disease is four times more common now than 60 years ago and affects about one in 100 people. According to Mayo studies, undiagnosed celiac disease can quadruple the risk of death. Mayo researchers are working to discover the causes and improve diagnosis.

In Barbara Tomen's July, 2012 article in *Discovery's Edge*, the Mayo Clinic's free online newsletter, Joseph Murray, M.D., a Mayo gastroenterologist and gluten specialist, writes about CD as a public health issue. Studies show four times the incidence of CD in 2012 as compared to 1950, with possible fatal complications if untreated.

In a subsequent study, Dr. Murray found that nearly half of celiac patients diagnosed during adulthood don't experience complete intestinal healing. A small proportion—not more than one in 50—has "refractory celiac disease" where the intestine doesn't improve at all after gluten is eliminated. "As many as half of those patients may be dead within three years," Dr. Murray says. "That's a rare condition, but one which we've been very invested in because that's the sharp end of celiac disease." Because of these findings, Mayo advocates greater vigilance in celiac cases. "It's not enough to say, 'You've got celiac disease, be gluten-free, goodbye,'" Dr. Murray says. "Celiac disease requires medical follow-up." I suggest finding a gluten nutritional expert and/or gastroenterologist and working together as a team with the doctor who diagnosed you.

The more people on the planet we want to feed, and the more willing we are to support chemical additives and artificial growth hormones in our food, the more the biochemical corporations profit. Whole Foods Market announced in 2012, that despite the FDA's resistance to pass a GMO labeling law in California, WFM would require all their food vendor manufacturers to declare GMO on their labels by 2018. According to varied media sources and employee interviews, however, WFM employees may have been trained to tell customers, when asked, that no products have GMO. Dangerous misinformation, especially for pregnant women and customers with celiac disease. In addition, the plastic that contains the labeled products is toxic!

Most countries in Europe and Asia don't buy U.S. corn and soy, because those two products are the most GMO-contaminated. As a result, our farmers are overstocked because of U.S. government subsidy deals. The government encourages evryone to eat more soy and corn, and tells us to do so through the media on a daily basis. More dangerous misinformation.

The bottom line is: If you value your health, beware of processed and packaged food and EAT REAL!

A bulletin from the Center for Food Safety announced September 27, 2013:

Victory! "Monsanto Protection Act" Killed in the Senate

After more than a year of fighting the biotech rider, dubbed the "Monsanto Protection Act," Senator Mikulski (D-MD) announced she was striking it from both the short-term continuing resolution (CR) to fund the government for the next 3 months, and that it is not in either the House or Senate 2014 appropriations bills! This is a huge victory. [...]

The "Monsanto Protection Act" was bad policy and had no place in a short-term spending bill. Removing it from the bill preserves the strength of our judicial review system and is a major win for the food movement.

Not only is GMO labeling a reasonable and common sense solution to the continued controversy that corporations like Monsanto, DuPont and Dow Chemical have created by subverting our basic democratic rights, but it is a basic right that citizens in 62 other countries around the world already enjoy, including Europe, Russia, China, India, South Africa and Saudi Arabia.

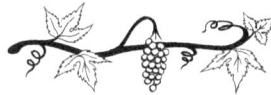

When I discovered I was gluten-sensitive, I had the usual reaction at first.

FEAR!

After a few days reflection, however, I was actually relieved to learn that I had a severe health challenge that I might be able to control. At that time, I jumped into the G-F diet with excitement and passion. After I eliminated all wheat, rye and barley—as well as sugar—from my diet, I felt better immediately, no tummy aches or mood swings, and much less anxiety.

Hallelujah! After years of searching for the cause of these and other symptoms, I had finally clarified my problems. I had less brain fog, my memory improved, and I had more energy. I began to lose weight even though I ate everything I wanted except gluten products and sugar. I lost 40 pounds easily in a short time, when no previous diets had ever worked for me. And the best thing was that I could eat as much as I wanted of vegetables and protein as often as I was hungry. No more frustration because I was always craving, as in the past—another of gluten's symptoms. This new gluten-free regime revolutionized my life.

Many of my cravings at the time were psychological and emotional, and my brain controlled my reactions. These cravings manifested as a hormone imbalance. I experienced all the other symptoms carried by any addiction such as heroin or alcohol. Because I wasn't completely successful at eliminating all the sugars in my diet, I was still an addict. One reason the gluten-free diet is so dangerous is because gluten-free products are processed and packaged with large amounts of sugar. Cravings will persist because the gluten must be replaced with protein and dark green vegetables and healthy fats, the proper amount of Omega-3s, and other essential vitamins and antioxidants. Emotionalism as another factor that influences our digestion. It is beneficial to learn to distinguish between emotions and feelings. When I feel what goes on inside and outside of my body, I balance my life and feel more of my gypsy freedom.

Byron Richards, the inspiring and knowledgeable doctor, has an online radio show, and his information about cravings is very valuable:

http:// www.wellnessresources.com/weight/articles
/digestive_inflammation_and_food_cravings/

It's not enough to guess about your own G-F health challenges, because any gluten challenge can affect your longevity. I am coming to terms of late with the idea that, in spite of the expense, I must do more detailed tests for vitamin and other deficiencies, such as the need for certain levels of EFAs and digestive enzymes.

I test on a regular basis for the basics, such as uric acid, cancer markets, blood sugar, and thyroid. Most health insurance, however, doesn't cover more in-depth and detailed tests. Healthy often presuppposes wealthy in a country without socialized medicine.

Since I began the hair analysis diet with personalized supplement plan, I feel new again!

Dr. Osborne continues to clarify the gluten intolerance issue:

> "True food allergies refer to foods that trigger the immune system to acutely produce massive amounts of the chemical histamine that leads to anaphylaxis. This potentially fatal condition causes the throat and esophagus to swell, cutting off air from the lungs, or may simply cause hives, skin rashes, and other non-life-threatening reactions."

See Dr. Osborne's website:

https://mail.google.com/mail/ca/u/0/?ui=2&ik=d13814b094&view=att
&th=13ae5c8bf1951afa&attid=0.1.1&disp=emb&zw&atsh=1

Once celiac disease, an autoimmune disease, has had an accurate diagnosis, it is easy to proceed toward symptom elimination. As of July 2013, however,

Dr. Osborne declared that he is the only doctor in the world who does the complete diagnosis to distinguish between CD, gluten sensitivity, and gluten intolerance. Dr. Osborne says other doctors only do two-thirds of the analysis, so they never get a perfect diagnosis. Many people, especially seniors, who have had the same basic diet for decades, are in denial about their eating habits. They don't want to change and don't know where and how to start the G-F regime.

Doctors appear hesitant to recommend this regime, possibly because they don't want to follow it themselves. Many in the medical and nutritional world consider that avoiding all grains is too complicated and unappetizing. Are they afraid to lose their clients if they recommend it and don't follow it themselves?

I learned through my own experience with gluten intolerance that we are all very unique when it comes to what we choose to eat and what we are willing to do to improve our health. After ten years on a G-F regime, I learn something new on a daily basis, both because of my own body's reactions to food intake and due to the daily research I do about gluten.

Gluten challenges can appear at any age and often become permanent. (I only discovered mine at age sixty-eight after many years of physical and emotional misery.) Symtoms are more frequent in women and affect both the digestive and neurological systems, as gluten attacks both the central and peripheral nervous tissue and causes deterioration. Some experts say gluten trauma is reversible. It definitely improves as long as you stay on the regime, but once I cheat the symptoms reoccur and take from a few days to a week to completely disappear. Sometimes I am affected by foods I eat outside of my home and don't suspect they contain gluten.

The statistics from a glutenology conference in Houston in March, 2013 suggest that it may take up to three years or more to heal from a gluten problem because of the thirty-year buildup that most people with a gluten challenge experience. That means commitment to a 100% gluten-free diet in the beginning—no risk-taking at restaurants, or dinners with family and friends. Either that or take your own food wherever you eat. Most of us are not willing to be that rigid, but this is the only way to deal with this issue at the present time.

There are more than 200 conditions that result from gluten challenges. Some conditions that can be related to gluten sensitivity and CD include the following:

Abdominal cramps, gas and bloating	Down's syndrome
ADHD/ADD	Epilepsy
Alcoholism	Foul-smelling or grayish stools (that may be fatty or oily)
Anemia	
Autism	Hepatitis C
Brain Fog	Iron deficiency
Chronic diarrhea of unknown origin	Microscopic colitis (inflammation of colon)
Chronic Fatigue and Fibromyalgia	Migraines
Colon Cancer	Mothers of kids w/ neural tube defects
Degenerative disc disease	Multiple Sclerosis
Dental & bone disorders (as osteoporosis)	Relatives of those with celiac disease or gluten-sensitive individuals
Depression	
Dermatitis herpetiformis	
Dermatomyositis	Unexplained rashes
Developmental Delays	Unexplained weight loss (or gain)
Diabetes mellitus	

Also, any autoimmune disease (common ones include):

Asthma	Muscle and joint pain
Brain fog	Muscle twitching
Cerebella ataxia (unexplained dizziness)	Nerve damage
Carpal Tunnel	Neuropathy
Dysbiosis	Osteoporosis
Dental defects	PCOS (Polycystic Ovarian Syndrome)
Failure to thrive (FTT) or short stature in children	
	Peripheral neuropathy
Female infertility (includes those with multiple miscarriages)	Psoriasis
	Psychiatric disorders (Schizophrenia and Bipolar)
Fatigue	
Gastresophageal reflux disease (GERD)	Rashes and skin diseases
Hashimoto's thyroiditis	Rheumatoid Arthritis
Inflammatory bowel disease	Scleroderma
Insomnia	Seizure disorders
Irritability	Jorgen's syndrome
IBS (Irritable Bowel Syndrome	Skin rash
Irritable bowel syndrome (IBS)	Stunted Growth in Children
Leaky Gut	Thyroid disease
Liver disease of unknown origin	Tingling in the legs and feet (Neuropathy)
Lupus	
Migraine Headaches	Tummy aches
Mouth sores	Weakness and Fatigue
Mood swings	Weight loss
Muscle cramps	

MayClinic Free Online Newsletter: *Discovery's Edge*, July 2010:

Irritability or depression
Anemia
Stomach upset
Joint pain
Muscle cramps
Skin rash
	Mouth sores
	Dental and bone disorders
	  (such as osteoporosis)
	
	Tingling in the legs and feet
	  (neuropathy)

In the *Wall St Journal*, 3/15/11, Melinda Beck observed that some indications of malabsorption of nutrients that may result from celiac disease include: Diarrhea or constipation, abdominal cramps, gas and bloating, general weakness and fatigue, foul-smelling or grayish stools that may be fatty or oily, stunted growth (in children), and osteoporosis.

Some experts think as many as one in 20 Americans may have some form of gluten sensitivity, but there is no test or defined set of symptoms. The most common are IBS-like stomach problems, headaches, fatigue, numbness and depression, but more than 200 other symptoms have been loosely linked to gluten intake, which is why it has been so difficult to study. Peter Green, director of the Celiac Disease Center says that research into gluten sensitivity today is roughly where celiac disease research was 30 years ago.

Gluten sensitivity comes from innate immunity, a primitive system with which the body sets up barriers to repel invaders. In a recent test, the subjects with celiac disease rallied by adaptive immunity, a more sophisticated system that develops specific cells to fight foreign bodies.

The findings still need to be replicated. How a reaction to gluten could cause such a wide range of symptoms also remains unproven. Dr. Fasano and other experts speculate that once immune cells are mistakenly primed to attack gluten, they can migrate and spread inflammation, even to the brain, which can result in glutenataxia.

Indeed, Marios Hadjivassiliou, a neurologist in Sheffield, England, says he found deposits of antibodies to gluten in autopsies and brain scans of some patients with ataxia, a condition of impaired balance.

Could such findings help explain why some parents of autistic children say their symptoms have improved—sometimes dramatically—when gluten was eliminated from their diets? To date, few scientific studies have emerged to

◆ HSP LIFEGUIDE

WHAT IS FOOD SENSITIVITY?

How does food sensitivity differ from gluten intolerance and classic food allergies?

Dr. Osborne explains in one of his informative videos:

"The inability to tolerate foods and environmental factors, also known as sensitivity or intolerance, induces chronic activation of the innate immune system and gives rise to inflammatory processes, which includes excess production of reactive oxygen species and the release of preformed and newly synthesized mediators of inflammation.

"This type of inflammation has been linked to countless chronic conditions, including: digestive disorders, migraines, obesity, chronic fatigue, ADD, aching joints, skin disorders, arthritis and many more."

For up-to-date information for HSPs about food sensitivity and gluten-intolerance, visit:

HighlySensitivePeople.com/gluten-free

back up such reports, although I know children with "ADD and ADHD" who lost their symptoms when they eliminated gluten from their diet.

Dr. Fasano hopes to eventually discover a biomarker specifically for gluten sensitivity. In the meantime, he and other experts recommend that anyone who thinks they have it be tested for celiac disease first. For now, a gluten-free diet is the only treatment recommended for gluten sensitivity, though some may be able to tolerate small amounts.

One of my favorite resources for my gluten research is the Gluten-Free Society's free *Ontology* newsletter and Dr. Peter Osborne's *Gluten-FreeWarrior.com*. His ontological information is documented and packed with valuable, cutting-edge information about the gluten intolerance, gluten sensitivity, and different allergy categories. His valuable videos and CDs advise how to deal with the gluten challenges in a simple and understandable way. He states that the only other quasi-definitive test for CD is the intestinal biopsy, which is more complicated and time consuming. Most tests for CD are not definitive, as sometimes the test will show negative because the gluten protein itself doesn't appear as the culprit, and the person is still challenged. Dr. Osborne has an explanation for this mystery on his informative and valuable website:

http://www.glutenfreesociety.org/video-tutorial /gluten-sensitivity-what-is-it/

Dr. Osborne's research studies are just another example of an infinite and ever-growing list of medical research that documents the existence of non-CD, gluten-related sensitivity. Why is this research important? Most doctors don't know the difference from the various ways gluten problems show up as allergies, sensitivities, intolerance, and/or CD.

NEUROLOGICAL DISORDERS CONNECTED WITH GLUTEN

Brain fog, tingling in the feet and hands, numbness sensations in your extremities, developmental delays, learning disabilities, as well as other symptoms such as Asperger's, autism, mitochondrial disorders, Tourette's, ataxia, depression, migraines and schizophrenia can all be related to gluten. Many doctors still don't connect the gluten issue with Crone's Disease, Irritable Bowel (IBS), Acid Reflux, or Leaky Gut, and don't understand the bottom line that they share—gluten in any form, when not tolerated by the digestive tract, causes inflammation to the immune system and decreases the metabolism's ability to function normally.

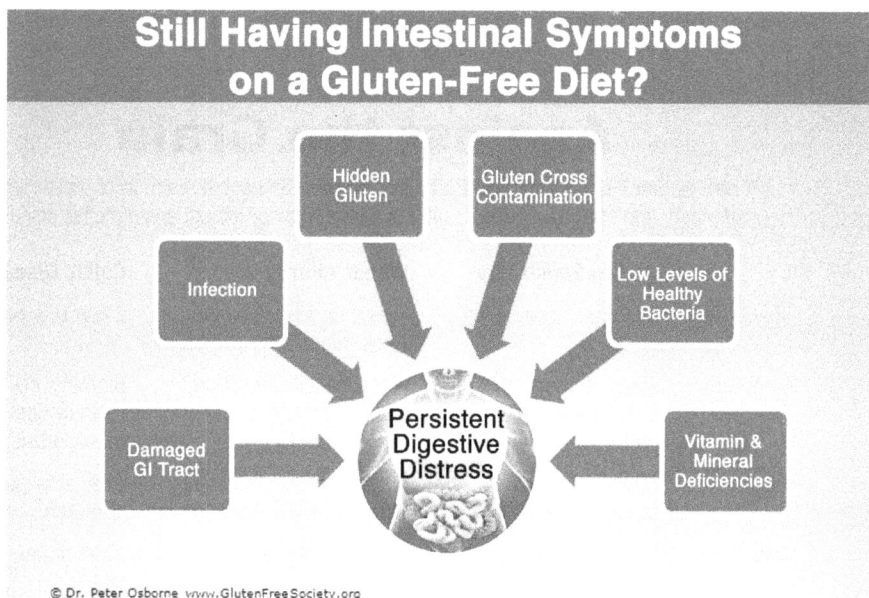

Still Having Intestinal Symptoms on a Gluten-Free Diet?

Hidden Gluten

Gluten Cross Contamination

Infection

Low Levels of Healthy Bacteria

Damaged GI Tract

Persistent Digestive Distress

Vitamin & Mineral Deficiencies

© Dr. Peter Osborne www.GlutenFreeSociety.org

BREAST-FEEDING AND GLUTEN

One recent article by Dr. Anna Kaplan, who retired to take care of her son who had severe food allergies and immune deficiency, shares that her son wasn't allergic to wheat, but because of his other allergies, he had allergic reactions to baked goods and many processed foods. Dr. Kaplan is on the advisory board of The Gluten Free Club (*www.glutenfreeclub.com*). In an 11/23/2012 article titled "Breast Feeding and Gluten," Dr. Kaplan shares that gluten is not filtered out from breast milk, and that all prospective mothers (even if they don't know if they have a gluten problem) should go on a gluten-free diet before they become pregnant and not add gluten until the infant is a few months old if at all.

Studies have been done worldwide on breast-feeding and gluten. Most modern doctors recommend that infants breastfeed for the first six months unless there is an actual danger to mother or baby that makes it impossible. Breastfed infants have their mother's antibodies, which protect them against infection, including the viral intestinal infections that are thought to be one possible trigger for CD.

Some of this information comes from an epidemic of celiac disease in young children that occurred in Sweden between 1984 and 1996. The diagnosis of

Against the Grain

A new research study indicates that some people can have a reaction to gluten even when they don't have any diagnosable wheat allergy or indications of celiac disease.

	Gluten Sensitivity	Wheat Allergy	Celiac Disease
Prevalence	6% of U.S. population	Less than 1% of children; some adults after exercise	1% of U.S. population
Symptoms	Some stomach issues, also headaches, balance problems, many others	Hives, nasal congestion, nausea, anaphylaxis	Bloating, diarrhea, malnutrition, osteoporosis; cancer
Triggers	Gluten (amount unknown)	Wheat proteins, but may cross-react with other grains	Even small amounts of gluten
Treatment	Gluten-free diet (small amounts may be tolerable)	Avoid wheat products	Strict gluten-free diet

Source: Wall Street Journal reporting

CD in children under two years of age was four times the usual amount. As the children born during these years were followed, three percent developed celiac disease by age 12. Those children who were breastfeeding with normal mothers at the time of gluten exposure had a lower risk of CD, as did those who continued to breastfeed after gluten was added to the diet.

Recommendations from some doctors for babies at risk for CD included breastfeeding, with gluten introduced into the diet between four and six months of age, and while breastfeeding continues, in order to minimize the risk of CD. One gluten expert recommend antibody testing for all mothers and three-year old children to offer a possible cure if the child's gluten challenge is detected early. But in short, all facts are not in about breast feeding and gluten-sensitive mothers.

Even though the USDA, the scientific and medical worlds, and the media have not done enough until recently to educate the public about the gluten challenge, there is a huge amount of information online. The documentation is often confusing. Check the resource section of this book and Google celiac forums. You will find solutions to your challenges through a grassroots movement to win the battle against gluten. Neighborhood support groups and online forums provide excellent support.

[1] *http://www.sott.net/article/224720-Scientists-have-discovered-that-Celiac-Disease-Can-be-the-Root-Cause-of-most-Neurological-Disorders*

5

MEAT

ILLUSTRATION BY E. MAZA, ARTIST

PRIMO PIATTO
(MAIN COURSE)

LAMB STEW WITH LEEKS AND BABY ARTICHOKES

SERVES 6

INGREDIENTS

3½ pounds boneless lamb shoulder meat, trim excess fat,
    cut into 2-inch pieces

1¼ cups chopped fresh Italian parsley

3 garlic cloves, minced

1 Tbsp. finely grated lemon peel

3 Tbsp. organic grapeseed oil

2 large leeks (white and pale green parts only), thinly sliced(about 2½ cups)

1 large onion, thinly sliced

¾ teaspoon fresh thyme, minced

1½ cups (or more) low-salt organic chicken broth

½ lemon

18 organic baby artichokes (about 1¾ pounds), prepared,
    or 1 package frozen artichoke hearts, or 1 can artichoke hearts.

1 Tbsp. olive oil

PREPARATION

Place trimmed lamb in large bowl; sprinkle generously with salt.
Cover and let stand at room temperature 30 minutes.

Combine 1 cup chopped parsley, minced garlic, and grated lemon
peel in small bowl. Reserve remaining ¼ cup parsley for garnish.

Heat oil in heavy large pot over high heat. Working in batches,
add lamb and cook until well browned on all sides, about
7 minutes per batch. Transfer lamb to medium bowl.

Add leeks and onion to drippings in pot and sauté until
softened, about 7 minutes. Add garlic, chopped parsley
mixture and thyme; stir 30 seconds.

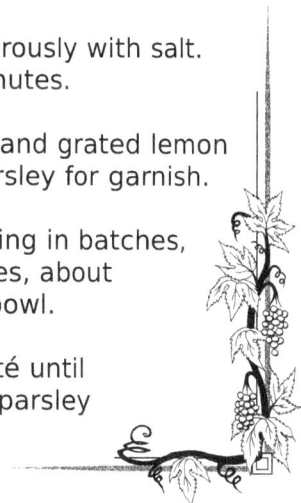

Return lamb and any accumulated juices to pot. Add 1½ cups broth and bring to boil. Reduce heat to medium-low, cover and simmer until lamb is very tender, about 1½ hours.

Add artichoke hearts: Cook fresh or frozen hearts for 10 minutes, or until tender. Add canned hearts for 5 minutes when lamb is tender.

Sprinkle with extra parsley, squeeze with fresh lemon, and drizzle with olive oil.

Lamb stew can be prepared one day ahead of serving. Cool slightly. Refrigerate stew uncovered until cold, then cover and keep refrigerated. Remove the excess fat. Bring lamb stew to a simmer before continuing with recipe to add parsley, lemon juice, and olive oil.

Fresh Artichokes
Fill medium bowl with cold water. Squeeze juice from lemon half into water; add squeezed lemon half. Break off tough outer leaves from one artichoke where leaves break naturally, stopping when first yellow leaves are reached.

Cut off stem and top ½ inch from artichoke, then cut artichoke in half lengthwise and drop into lemon water. Repeat with remaining artichokes.

Drain artichokes and add to lamb stew. Bring to boil. Reduce heat to medium-low, cover, and simmer until artichokes are tender, adding more broth by ¼ cupful if stew is dry, about 25 minutes.

Season stew to taste with salt and pepper flakes. Transfer to bowl; sprinkle lamb stew with reserved ¼ cup chopped parsley and drizzle with olive oil.

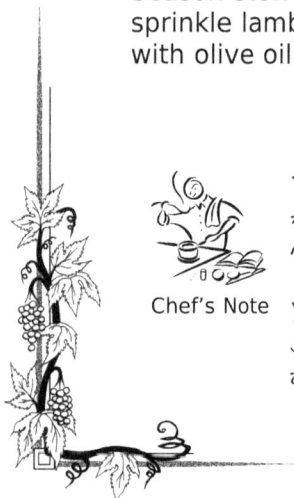

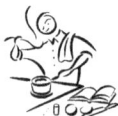

Chef's Note

To save time, have the butcher trim the excess fat from the lamb shoulder and cut the meat into two-inch pieces

You can add 1 cup red or white wine after sautéing the lamb, and reduce before adding the artichokes.

MEAT AND ME

Red meat has been my favorite food all my life. My mother hated to cook, and I grew up on steaks, chops, and some frozen veggies. When I first married, Massimo and I were invited to the home of a very wealthy and distinguished Italian admiral and his wife for dinner with other high-ranking naval military personnel, all very elegant in their uniforms, embellished with various glittery gold braid and other decorations. A formal dinner party on the terrace of an elegant Roman apartment was an honored invitation for Americans and Italians alike. Our sophisticated and beautiful hostess served thick, rare, juicy Bistecca Fiorentina. The Italians don't feed their cattle GMO and their best beef, the Chianina, is always grass-fed. In fact, American breeders have begun to interbreed them with other cattle breeds for lower fat and enhanced taste.

The T-bone steak cut is a Florentine invention Catherine de Medici introduced to France and dates from the 1500s or before. The tastiest part of any meat is the bone, and I was always favored with the steak bones at my family's dinner table. I mentioned this in a casual way to my host, the admiral, as I saw everyone had left their bones untouched.

He jumped up immediately and announced that I must chew my own bone right on the spot. I took the challenge, tied my napkin around my neck, and ate the bone with great satisfaction, as the more conservative guests glanced at each other with shocked expressions. I was satisfied I had cemented the reputation that Americans had at the time of being a *pazza straniera*—a crazy foreigner.

I didn't mention I was disappointed in the flavor. My 3-inch thick, beautiful T-bone steak lacked the taste its appearance promised. I later learned that I was used to GMO corn and soy fed beef, (GMO for cattle began in the fifties when I was growing up), and the grass-fed Chianina had less fat and chemicals so it tasted more bland and was a more authentic taste my palate no longer recognized.

WHAT IS MEAT?

According to Wikipedia, "Red meat is darker-colored meat, as contrasted with white meat. Exact definition varies by time, place, and culture, but the meat of adult mammals such as cows, buffalo, lamb, goat, sheep, horse, ducks, geese, and wild game is invariably considered red."

When I began this book I was uncertain about whether I should continue to eat meat. I researched a variety of articles and books, because I wanted to write with an unbiased approach about meat and vegetarianism. I thought meat was best for me, but what about everyone else?

WHY MEAT?

There is a great deal of controversy and confusion today about whether "to meat or not to meat." I am partial to grass-fed buffalo that has not been finished before slaughter with corn and soy, as is often the practice with so-called "grass-fed beef" and "pastured chickens." I have researched the issue for my own clarity and peace of mind as well as to inform my readers so they can make their best choice on the topic. I went vegetarian for a few months when I was in my forties. When I researched that diet more because I didn't feel as energetic as I wanted to, I read about my blood type and saw that because my ancestors ate meat, I should eat red meat. I needed the B-12, especially as I was getting older. So, I began to explore the Paleo Diet, which is based on protein and vegetables, before grain cultivation began.

Irma Jennings, Holistic Bone Coach, founder of Food for Healthy Bones, in her blog, *http://www.food4healthybones.com/blog/*, writes:

> "Grain-fed beef, on the other hand, is high in Omega-6 fats. They're also necessary for good health but Omega-6s are stiffer, and promote blood clotting and inflammation. And as Dr. Oz would tell you, inflammation is the root of all chronic disease. A healthy balance of Omega-3s to Omega-6s is 1:1, equal amounts of each. Unfortunately, the average American consumes 40 times more Omega-6s than Omega-3s. That imbalance has led to our epidemic of chronic diseases including heart disease, cancer, asthma, arthritis, and depression."

Irma asks, "Why are we so out of balance with our Omega-3 and Omega-6?"

> "One reason is our meat supply. When you feed cows grass, their meat contains more Omega-3s. But when you feed them corn and soy their meat contains more Omega-6s. In fact, grain-fed beef has 10 times more Omega-6s than Omega-3s. But grass-fed/grass-finished beef comes very close to the perfect 1:1 ratio for human health."

(Permission granted from Irma to use her quote.)

As a marketing coach for creative entrepreneurs, gluten expert, author, lecturer, consultant, chef and cooking teacher, I receive many questions about meat when I consult with celiacs and other people who want to design their "perfect diet." To be more specific, when I write about "Meat" in this book, in the main part, I refer to beef — red meat — which many people relate to in an animalistic way — bloody, raw, overcooked, undercooked or cooked to perfection, tender or tough, chewy, tender, gristly or smooth, red, pink, brown, gray, substantial, energizing, foraging, beefy, fiber (as in moral fiber), fat, rich, a tasty morsel, branded, buttery, tough, beefing it up, tough fiber, muscle, hunk, red-blooded, beastly, and bovine — all words which both meat eaters and those who would never touch meat use to describe red meat.

Humanity has created a story about beef, which has been transmuted to other symbolic and descriptive meanings in the English language, as well as in many romance languages. Many of the past U.S. marketing tag lines were international clichés like Wendy's "Where's the Beef?" and their "If Angus be Music, Rock On."

I want to clarify the meat industry's industrialization issue for you and present some myths and realities around this controversial subject. Meat is a very important cultural phenomenon, not just a food product. Different religions and cultures treat beef according to their own bias. People in the U.S. crave and consume millions of hamburgers daily, yet the Jain sect of India worships the cow and is forbidden to consume even one bite of red meat. As Nick Fiddes writes in his book, *Meat: A Natural Symbol,*

> "A moral and ideological judgment and an economic reference point can also be associated with what we eat. Today, the more affluent and better educated eat less meat than in the past, (the poor eat more, even though some must cut their budget in other areas to eat it more frequently), for a variety of reasons, most due to philosophy, religion, and ecological biases."

Red meat is a protein that builds strong bones and flexibility. Adults need about 50 grams of protein a day. Four ounces of red meat has about 28 grams of protein. I recommend to eat a portion the size of your palm. This goes for babies, too, as they have very small tummies and don't need large quantities of anything. We all need the vitamin B-12, especially as we age, and it is more easily absorbed through red meat than in any other way.

PINK SLIME

All countries and religions have different meanings and values associated with meat — after all, the history of meat eaters and hunters is five million years old. America has an extrinsic meat industry, where most livestock is not raised in pastures but in feedlots, and fattened with GMO corn, soy and antibiotics. This extrinsic, industrialized beef from animals raised in *confined animal feeding operations* (CAFOs) contains large quantities of antibiotics and other toxins. Discarded manure that contains toxins, such as pesticides and antibiotics, infects rivers and our drinking water, killing fish, algae, and other living organism (as do our human medical products when not disposed of properly).

According to the website *pinkslime.com*, in late 2011 and early 2012 the food safety topic caught the attention of celebrity chefs (such as Jamie Oliver), the media, and the public, and the furor arose. In an investigative report by ABC News in early 2012, it was discovered that approximately 70% of all ground beef sold in grocery stores and supermarkets contained pink slime. One fast-food hamburger often has as many as 100 different cows ground into the patty with chemical fillers. Shortly thereafter, many restaurants stopped buying pink slime ground beef. Grocery store and supermarket chains started banning pink slime meat, and some school districts stopped buying pink slime products for their cafeterias.

MEAT AND ME

I don't prescribe my personal diet for my readers. I created my personal food plan over more than fifty years and was a red meat eater all my life with periodic breaks to try a variety of diets. The Paleo diet suits me well: Animal protein, greens, nuts, and seeds. I eat a fist-size portion of red meat twice a week at the most. I avoid gluten in any form. Some experiments, such as vegetarianism and macrobiotics, worked for me for a few years then eventually failed. Others, such as the gluten-free, succeeded later on. I have learned that my diet must change as I evolve.

I now eat buffalo or grass-fed beef once a week and small fish, raw organic horsemeat, ostrich and goat, which I wish were more available in the U.S., as they are in much of Italy and other parts of Western Europe. My local

Whole Foods Market now carries some game and goat, and I sometimes buy wild boar at the Asian market. Specialty meats are available online, but they are expensive. I also buy my grass-fed, organic beef at the farmers market from Novy Organics.

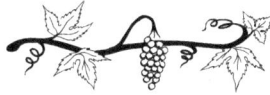

As an 18-year-old art student in 1958, I was fortunate to experience one of Man's first graphic portrayals of his relationship to meat. I was transfixed while studying the symbols of ancient cattle, bison and deer drawn in charcoal and blood on the cave walls of Lascaux and Altamira, before they were closed off due to deterioration from moisture from people's breath. These graceful and touching animal symbols were painted 17,000 years ago during the Middle Paleolithic Stone Age.

For hundreds of years, art historians and anthropologists have struggled to decipher the meaning of these prehistoric symbols with no agreement. Are they religious? Spiritual? Inspirational? Celebrations of courage and victory? Ritualistic? Dietary recommendations? A combination of all these and more? Certain anthropologists theorize that women granted sex as an incentive to the hunter who "brought home the most mastodon bacon," while some art historians believe they honored the animals they hunted by painting sacred symbols on their cave walls. Although experts may disagree on Neanderthal social and spiritual practices, one thing is clear — our paleo ancestors were definitely carnivores. And despite all our technological and scientific advances, we have not evolved a new digestive tract for grains.

Whatever the precise meaning these ancient, beautiful and touching portrayals hold, I can relate to the link that exists over the many thousands of years and the important relationship to meat that I and many other humans experience, even though we may not always be conscious of how we are connected. For example, in the same area of the Dordogne as the Lascaux caves, a modern-day rancher attempts to resuscitate the huge, ancient Aurochs breed. They are descended from and resemble the cave painting cattle of the Paleolithic age. The meat is supposed to be tender and tasty. When it is available commercially, I would like to taste it.

MEAT AND NUTRITION

The Greeks defined proteins with the word *protos*, which means "first." Proteins consist of molecules called amino acids, the basic building blocks of the human body. We have 25 different amino acids in one protein molecule. Our cells and DNA use protein, as well as enzymes and hormones, to build muscles and bones, as well as hair and fingernails. All of these nutrients are absorbed by our small intestines to be transported in the bloodstream. Gluten is a protein, as well. If the villi of the intestine become flattened because of wheat and gluten sensitivities, they are no longer able to absorb these nutrients, and we risk anemia and other life threatening diseases.

Meat in small quantities is easier for most of us to digest than grains, as it doesn't convert to sugar. When I eat a fistful of organic, rare, grass-fed red meat or organic calves or chicken liver, I feel immediately energized from the B-12. I also enjoy the Buffalo Clod cut sliced very thin and rare, or New Zealand natural lamb (no antibiotics), once a week.

As of 2010, almost 25% of our total fat consumption in the West is derived from meat and meat products, with an average consumption of three times weekly. The fat content of lean, red meat has fallen by an average of 30%. Only half of that fat is saturated. Buffalo contains mono-saturated fat, which is much healthier, but very dry. So some ranchers have started to add buffalo fat to the ground buffalo to increase the taste. Both beef and buffalo are more tender and tastier with a bit of fat. I hope buffalo ranchers don't begin to add GMO corn and soy to finish their product as most of the cattle ranchers do.

The general misconception about animal fat and high cholesterol still abounds. Some animal fat is actually good for us because it is high in Omega-3s, an essential necessity for good health. The meat is tastier and more tender with some fat. When red meat is consumed with vegetables such as Italian kale, it helps the body absorb plant sources of minerals such as copper, chromium, zinc, selenium and iron. It also prevents anemia and helps to maintain the nervous system. Soups are the best way to absorb nutrients, because they are more easily digestible. Four ounces of red meat supplies 16% of the recommended daily intake of iron.

I also take vitamin B-12 injections, because many older people do not absorb B-12 in supplement form. We all need B-12, especially seniors and anemics. Both my MD and naturopathic nutritionist recommend a couple of small servings of red meat a week to have my best energy. Beef contains the nutrients: iron, zinc, selenium, vitamin B-12, creatine, phosphorous, niacin, thiamin, riboflavin, copper, alpha lipoic acid, and many other minerals. Prolonged protein deficiency may result in irreversible nerve damage and anemia.

Older people are often low in vitamin B-12, which can often affect the brain and cause memory loss. Eating red meat regularly is the most effective way to ensure you have enough. Red meat is one of the few sources of vitamin B-12 and vitamin K, which become harder to absorb through other foods as we age and can often result in anemia. The next best way to get enough of quality Vitamin B-12 is from substances such as bee pollen and royal jelly; however, they are expensive.

We can reduce the U.S. out-of-the-ballpark, trillion-dollar cost of healthcare by taking responsibility for our nutritional health. The government, media, and international corporations have their own issues around our diets. I prefer to research my best food choices myself, or consult a nutritionist, rather than follow the FDA's food pyramid advice. It doesn't work for me, because it is grain-based and is constantly changing. As a gluten-sensitive woman, I consider the amount of carbs the U.S. government recommends a threat to my health and longevity. "Across the Board" diets are dangerous, and I recommend each person research his own or consult a qualified nutritionist who knows about gluten and don't depend exclusively on the FDA.

We need to do our own research about our dietary needs with the help of expert nutritional experts and not depend on the government.

In *Newsweek* magazine, November 29, 2010, in an article titled "The Dinner Divide," Lisa Miller wrote: "Modern America is a place of extremes, and what you eat for dinner has become the definitive marker of social status." The richest Americans want offal when they dine out today — a far cry from the 1950s, when people in my hometown of Denver were shocked if someone ate garlic and olive oil, much less kidneys or sweetbreads. Due to the economic collapse of the 1980s, innards, which are very healthy for us when organic and contain no GMO and when harvested from grass-fed animals, are all the rage with cutting-edge chefs and restaurants around the world.

Nutritional expert Dr. Alfredo Urso, PhD says, "When intuition and science come together, many things are possible." Dr. Urso (*www.rejuvenateyourbody.net*)

is an Italian researcher who has spent thirty years to develop the Seven Nourishing Foundations theory. He and other experts proclaim that we can get all the nutrition we need, and absorb it with more ease, when we eat close to the Paleo diet, as ancient Neanderthals did: raw grass-fed meat, eggs, fish, chicken, green juice, organic soaked nuts and organic seeds, some organic fruits, bee pollen, coconut, Terramin clay for minerals, and seasoned with quality salt.

I feel better at age 77 than I have at any other time in my long life.

MEAT AND MORALS

The moral issue of whether or not to eat meat is entirely a personal decision. I am not against vegetarians, vegans or even the use of macrobiotics. In fact,

I respect vegetarians and vegans because many want to protect the animal kingdom from violence. Yet for many people, eating meat is perfectly acceptable. For example, the Native American religion teaches that animals are very grateful to sacrifice themselves in the hope of reincarnation as a human.

What I do strongly believe is that diet needs to be taken as a very important health issue, and each person needs to understand their inner self, their environment, their financial resources,

◆ HSP LIFEGUIDE

EAT WHEAT, MEAT AND DON'T SPURN THAT TREAT

Although important to be alert to sensitivities and avoid excess, *Highly Sensitive People* often do have a tendency to get carried away and sometimes become too rigid in their diet to the extent of neglecting to get adequate nutrition, especially protein and an occasional "splurge." Not only is variety in your nutritional habits good to maintain optimum health, it improves your morale!

And be sure you are eating enough protein daily. Some symptoms of protein deficiency that merit particular attention:

- Thinning hair
- Weak fingernails
- Poor digestion
- Muscle weakness
- Weakened heart

Even more serious are long-term effects such as fluid retention and stomach bloat.

For up-to-date information for HSPs about helpful nutritional practices and food sensitivities, visit:

HighlySensitivePeople.com/gluten-free

and their taste buds. You may also find it helpful to consult an expert nutritionist. Ideally, I want each person to take responsibility for their own health, to read labels carefully, and to call the manufacturer with any questions — don't take the food pyramid or the media's recommendations as the only truth. Research what you are eating and its origins online, and buy organic or from local farmers markets when possible. Avoid processed, packaged foods because of the toxins. Optimally, you may want to become a Locavore or grow your own.

Barbara Kingsolver recounts in her amazing and inspiring book, *Animal, Vegetable, and Miracle*, how she moved from Manhattan with her husband and two daughters to Kentucky, where they made a pact to only eat what they could grow. She succeeded in less time than she thought possible, even though they had to trade some produce and buy some organic products at farmers markets.

Another amazing book, called *The River Cottage Meat Book*, by the English chef and food writer Hugh Fearnley-Whittingstall, inspires me with other questions about moral and ethical content in the way we deal with the animals that provide us with meat. He says that Man has eaten meat for hundreds of thousands of years, and has only domesticated animals for tens of thousands of years. He adds that gorillas and orangutans are vegetarians, but chimps, the genetically closest to humans, eat meat and sometimes kill other monkey and chimp species.

MODERN MAN AND GRAINS

Scott Adams, Owner of the Gluten-Free Mall, was diagnosed with Celiac Disease in 1994. In 1995 he developed the Gluten-Free Mall web site (*www.celiac.com*) and online store with the blessings of the Celiac Organization. His free site offers the latest scientific research on gluten intolerance and the gluten challenge:

> "Gluten intolerance is strongly linked to specific genetic markers which have indeed required thousands years to develop and be selected: the 'population genetic' time is of this dimension, while the changes in the environment and in the food we eat, require centuries or less....Human beings have been on Earth for over 3 million years, but Homo sapiens, our nearest parent, is only 100,000 years old. For 90,000 years he

conducted a nomadic life getting food by hunting, fishing and collecting fruits, seeds, herbs and vegetables from nature. Only quite recently (about 10,000 years ago) did some nomadic tribes start to have stable settlements because they developed the ability to gather enough food to be stored. The cultivation of wild seeds began at that time."

Due to this cultivation, wild wheat was gathered and eventually domesticated. Wheat is a comparatively new grain and our digestive systems, which are still the same as those of the Neanderthals, are not able to digest wheat and many other grains with ease. It's a case of social development moving ahead of our biological evolution:

> "The discovery in the Neolithic age of ways to produce and store food has been the greatest revolution mankind ever experienced. Passage from collection to production originates the first system in which human labor is transferred onto activities, which produced income for long periods of time. The principle of property was consolidated and fortifications to protect the land and food stores were developed."

The Neanderthals ate whatever meat they could kill. Meat eating was a survival, spiritual, and ritualistic activity for the Neanderthal hunters and meat eaters. As we mentioned earlier, they ate whatever they could kill and gave honor to the animal as they painted the Aurochs, bear, and deer symbols on their sacred cave walls seen in Lascaux, France and Altamira, Spain. Most modern historians and archeologists interpret these bison and deer drawings and paintings as a kind of prayer: to bring hunters the courage and worthiness to nourish their spirit and tribe with this sacred meat.

I have an O blood type. My Russian and Western European ancestors were meat eaters, and I was brought up on steaks and chops from corn-fed beef, as well as red meat from duck, lamb, elk, and venison. My bloodline is formed from meat eaters—no vegetarians that I have ever heard of in my modern ancestry. My health and palate is satisfied with a serving of organic, grass-fed meat that averages about $1.50 a serving. Cattle that graze on mixed grasses in organic pastures as a steady diet from birth to slaughter is delicious and has no toxins.

Many U.S. ranchers, however, raise their cattle in pastures but finish them before slaughter with GMO wheat, oats, soy fodder, additives and growth hormones. GMO-fed beef is more difficult to digest than plants and grains, and contains arachidonic acid, an inflammatory substance that increases skin

NaturalNews — 6/16/2013 Recent announcements about the acquisition of U.S.-based Smithfield Foods Inc., the world's largest pork producer and processor, by a major Chinese holding company has sent significant shockwaves throughout the American economy. According to news reports, Shuanghui International Holdings Ltd. is in the process of pulling the trigger on purchasing Smithfield for $4.72 billion, a move that some say marks the beginning of a much larger takeover of American industry by the Far East.

Reports of a potential Smithfield acquisition have been surfacing here and there in recent months. But now it appears that the decision is all but complete, pending approval from Smithfield's shareholders. As reported by *Newsday.com*, the deal was officially announced at the end of May, and part of its terms included shareholders receiving $34 per share, a roughly 31 percent premium from earlier share value, as part of the deal.

The U.S. Committee on Foreign Investment still has to review the deal to assess any potential national security risks. But by the way the mainstream media is currently talking about the deal, it is essentially already a reality, which means a major segment of the American food economy will soon be controlled by a Chinese corporation. And not surprisingly, many of those paying attention to this development are completely outraged.

"There is public unease when a foreign buyer acquires the largest pork-producing company in the world that is a major player in the local economy and is the source of our bacon and ribs," wrote Sharon Valentine in a recent editorial published by *FayObserver.com*.

Source: http://www.naturalnews.com/040805_China_Smithfield_Foods_food_safety.html

disease symptoms and anemia. Inoculations are given to prevent or cure disease. If cows are not slaughtered pre-maturity they become very sick from these antibiotics they are fed. They become toxic over a period of time and die.

Kudos to Deborah Garcia, who produced the video *The Future of Food*, about Monsanto and GMO. Another video, *King Korn*, exposes the story that cows fed on Monsanto's GMO soy and corn must be slaughtered six months before they reach maturity. The GMO grains would kill them, as they are so indigestible when taken as a steady diet for cattle. The corn must be flaked or livestock won't touch it.

Cattle are often butchered by thoughtless and uncaring methods resulting in a more acidic taste due to the adrenaline created by the cattle's fear at slaughter, as well as GMO feed, antibiotics and other toxins. We end up eating and absorbing these toxins and stress hormones, which can result in kidney problems and gout.

We cook the meat in the same way primitive man did — on the grill, and we consume the carcinogens that develop through this ancient style of cooking meat.

Restaurants serve huge portions of beef, as heart disease in wealthier nations around the globe continues to rise. Some authorities believe large amounts of red meat can lead to certain cancers: breast, colon, stomach, lymphoma, bladder, prostate, and colorectal.

A *Time Magazine* article of February 2, 2011 titled "Where's The Beef?" reports that a beefy Five-Layer Burrito from Taco Bell has 560 calories and 23 grams of fat, for just 99 cents, 40% of which is chemical filler, labeled as "Taco Seasoning." Those 3-inch thick Rib eye steaks fed on GMO corn and soy also contribute to the pot bellies many acquire in their thirties.

I agree smaller quantities of red meat are best.

Modern herbalists, dieticians, and nutritionists evolved from the pre-historic women and men who were the doctors of their time — herbalists, and root gatherers who evolved into more scientific realms. Much of modern medicine is due to their experimentation and documentation.

MEAT AND TOXICITY

One piece of important information I learned from the August, 2010 issue of *Readers Digest Magazine* was in an article written by Michael Crouch, who wrote: "Some companies pump carbon monoxide into packaging to keep meat from turning brown. It is essential to check the label for additives. Despite the label 'Natural,' meat is often injected with sodium-like broth, salt water, or seaweed extract." I have learned to make a shopping list and take plenty of time to shop, so I can be certain to read the label before I buy anything at all and call the manufacturer with any questions.

Here's some information from Gaia-Health about this issue:
http://www.gaia-health.com/articles201/000226-usda-trashes-organic-pasture
-not-required-for-cows-last-4-months.shtml

Recently, I was amazed to learn that, although the FDA creates the rules and regulations around food safety, many times they will pass the regulation on a food product and omit the label, such as with GMO farmed fish, a regulation the FDA passed in August, 2010. In the general election of November 6, 2012, I voted for Proposition #37 which would require food products to tell me if there was any GMO in the food I was thinking about buying. To my dismay, that law was to pass in 2006 and didn't pass as a government law until August 2013. I am very grateful for the ruling; however, I will wait to see how detailed the labeling is and what the results are for infractions.

In March, 2013, Whole Foods announced that by 2018 all their products would be labeled. That is a commendable first step towards serving their customers with healthier food products. However, it doesn't address the fact that the packing itself is toxic. EAT REAL!

In Dr. Mercola's newsletters, (*www.mercola.com*), Tom Paine, reported in 2011 that the American Medical Association (AMA) had recently called for an end to the routine use of antibiotics in agriculture. Paine added, "With the Food and Drug Administration (FDA) unwilling or unable, to act, our medical arsenal is rapidly being depleted of one of its chief weapons in the fight against food-borne illness. A report by the Union of Concerned Scientists estimates as much as 70 percent of all antibiotics sold in the U. S. are fed to chickens, cattle and hogs — not to treat disease but to make the animals grow faster to slaughter more quickly for more profit. This increases profit margins for livestock producers, but it puts YOUR health at risk." The repeated use of antibiotics produces the need for stronger antibiotics because the viruses become resistant very quickly.

Eating organically may not entirely alleviate this problem, since organic crops, which cannot be fertilized with synthetic fertilizers, are the ones most often fertilized with manure. As it stands, manure that contains antibiotics is still allowed under the organic label. So it all depends on where the organic farmer gets his manure and what it contains. Some organic crop farmers may be getting their manure from organic cattle farms, but there's no guarantee that's taking place. The only way to find out is to ask the farmer first-hand.

Taking all of these factors into consideration, is it any wonder that the ratio of good-bacteria-to-bad is upside down in most people in our society?

The rise of antibiotic-resistance in livestock is so alarming that government officials have finally admitted you can become infected when you eat or simply handle infected meat. In a remarkable move by the current administration, the FDA is proposing to phase out antibiotics used to promote animals' growth. They also warn that the microbes can contaminate kitchen counters, utensils and other food. Mad Cow Disease is not a fairytale. There are still cases reported in the U.S. and England in 2013.

Food Democracy Now! believes that family farmers have a right to farm without threat and intimidation. We don't think farmers should be sued because Monsanto's patented genes from a neighbor's field blow across their fence and contaminate their organic or conventional, non-GMO seeds. That's why Monsanto is being sued in court to protect family farmers from unwanted genetic contamination of their crops and from Monsanto's abusive lawsuits.

Let's speed up the overhaul of regulation. Food Democracy Now! has created a petition against the overuse of antibiotics in livestock production.

HSP LIFEGUIDE

MORE RESEARCH OPTIONS

Below are some U.S. food agencies to contact for research and questions:

FDA Meat and Poultry Hotline
800-332-4010

FDA Seafood Hotline
800-332-4010

USDA Meat and Poultry Hotline
888-674-6854
mphotline.fsis@usda.gov

USDA Information Hotline
202-720-2791

Food Democracy Now
917-968-7369
dave@fooddemocracynow.org

FSIS
202-720-9113
tjosh.stull@fsis.usda.gov

NACMPI
NACMPI@fsis.usda.gov

For up-to-date information for HSPs about nutrition and further research links, visit:

HighlySensitivePeople.com/gluten-free

I urge you to visit their website, *www.fooddemocracynow.com*, and add your vote against the use of antibiotics and GMO used to raise livestock and agricultural.

POULTRY & GMO

Mercola, in the 1/14/2013 issue of his free newsletter, writes about "Latest Study Shows Roundup Creates Botulism Breeding Ground in Poultry." The article highlights a new German study from the Institute of Bacteriology and Mycology that states that Monsanto's chemical glyphosate affects poultry gut microbes. "Researchers found that highly pathogenic bacteria resisted glyphosate, whereas beneficial bacteria likely succumbed to it."

What does this mean for you and me? The essential implication is that poultry fed GE corn or soy would fall victim to dysbiosis, meaning unhealthy changes in their gut flora that threaten the health of the birds, as well as anyone consuming them. The good bacteria in the poultry gut such as *Enterococcus*, *Bifidobacterium* and *Lactobacillus* are killed off, allowing the pathogenic or disease-causing bacteria to flourish. Chickens bred in CAFOs are already routinely fed antibiotics, arsenic, and even antidepressants, all of which have serious adverse health consequences.

The implications of this become even clearer when you consider the recently released findings of a study that showed "GE feed can cause significant changes in the digestive systems, immune systems, and major organs (including liver, kidneys, pancreas, genitals and others) of rats, mice, pigs and salmon as a major threat to your health."[1]

All these chemicals contribute to the destruction of the planet's topsoil and contaminate the air and water, which leaves humans no sustainable survival resources.

Kelly at her blog site *www.Gluten-free labels.com* markets labels that are great for your kitchen. I also love to give them as gifts and put them on my homemade food gifts to support and educate. She writes on her blog that deli meats are sometimes gluten-free, but many are not. Even if it is labeled as such, there is still the issue of cross-contamination. Kelly suggests that gloves should be changed in meat departments, and the slicer should be wiped clean for gluten-sensitive customers. She adds that some brands offer small packages that are pre-cut and packaged in the meat department to avoid cross-contamination.

6

THE FAMILY MEAL

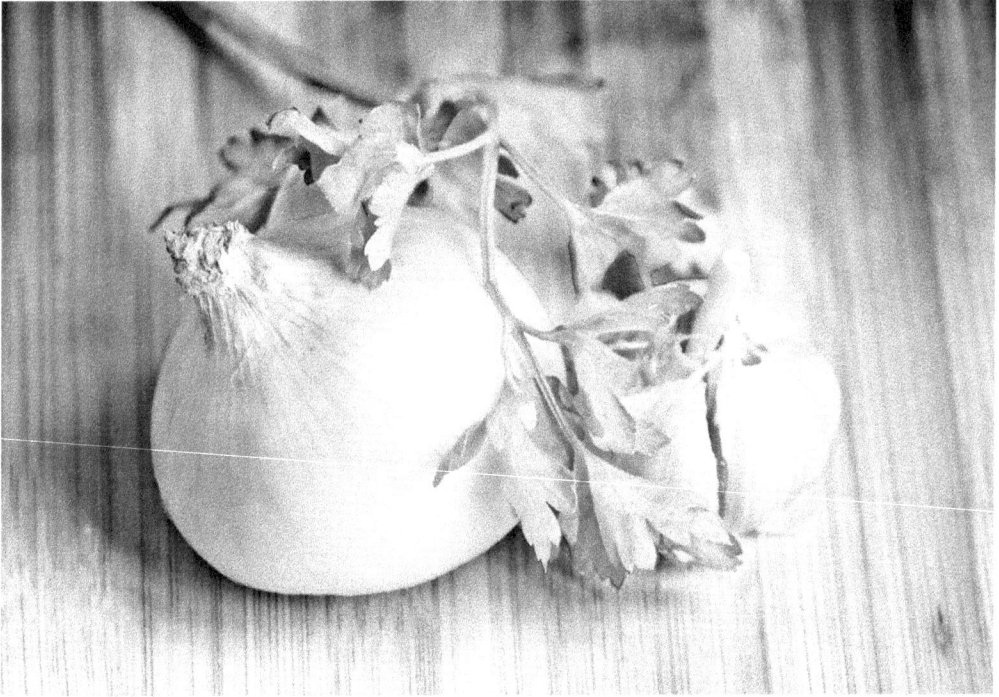

ANCORA PRIMO

Two for One!

Make a big pot of this soup and refrigerate overnight to remove fat from the broth. Freeze the leftover broth in small batches. The lesso rifatto stew is made from the soup ingredients and is a favorite with my Florentine family. Perfect for a cold winter night and to use as speedy backup dinners. The stew name means "Boiled and Remade." Use organic, non-GMO, grass-fed beef or buffalo, and pastured, soy and corn-free capon or chicken.

BEEF SOUP AND LESSO RIFATTO STEW

SERVES 6

INGREDIENTS

2½ pounds grass-fed organic beef or buffalo (shank, tongue, and other parts for boiling)

2 beef or buffalo shin bones

One-half organic capon or boiling chicken (optional)

1 organic whole onion

5 cloves organic garlic

2 organic carrots, peeled and cut into 3-inch lengths

1 organic celery stalk, chopped

1 cup fresh organic tomatoes, diced, or 1 can organic tomatoes, diced

½ cup organic Italian parsley, chopped

1 Tbsp. Himalayan salt

PREPARATION

Place all the ingredients in a large soup pot, and cover with pure water. Bring to a slow boil, covered for 1 hour. Skim the surface. Add the chicken and cook for another hour.

The beef should be very tender; the skin will easily come off the tongue. (I like to make this the night before so I can remove any excess fat from the broth.)

Remove the beef and vegetables from the broth. Discard the tomato parsley, and beef bones.

Strain the broth and replace the beef in the broth.

Reheat the beef and chicken and serve cut and arranged on a serving plate, with salt, extra virgin olive oil, mustard, and salsa verde.

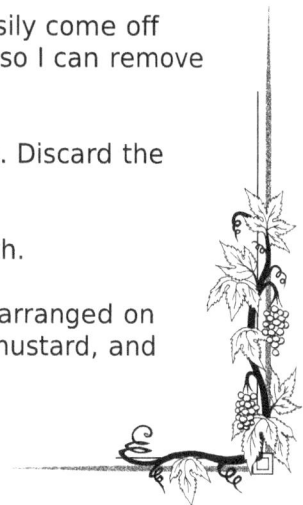

Salsa Verde

INGREDIENTS

1 cup organic Italian parsley, chopped
2 Tbsp. organic capers
3 garlic cloves, chopped
2 anchovy filets
Organic apple cider vinegar to taste
½ cup organic olive oil
½ cup organic pine nuts

PREPARATION

Mince or process the parsley, capers, garlic, anchovy, and pine nuts.

Put the mixture into a serving bowl and add olive oil and vinegar.

LESSO RIFATTO

INGREDIENTS

1 pound leftover boiled meat, chopped into small cubes
1½ pounds organic red onions, finely sliced
2 cups organic, diced tomatoes, or organic red wine
½ cup organic grape seed oil
1 Tbsp. fresh rosemary, chopped
1 Tbsp. organic olive oil
1 cup Italian parsley, chopped
Himalayan salt

PREPARATION

Sauté the onions in grape seed oil; when golden, add tomatoes or red wine. Season to taste with salt.

Bring to a boil and simmer for 10 minutes. Add the leftover beef and cook covered for an additional 20 minutes.

Add olive oil and parsley, and serve warm.

Chef's Note

Mince the meat and vegetables and add an egg and gluten-free breadcrumbs to make little patties or meatballs with the leftovers.

When you make the lesso rifatto, add some minced sage to the pan with the onions. Add bitter greens such as kale or Swiss chard.

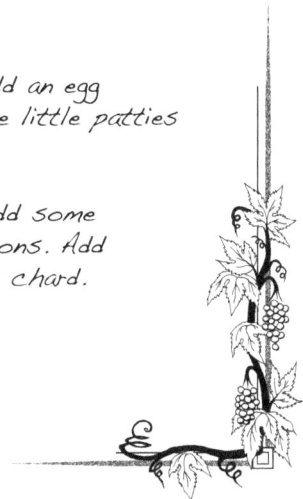

*I*n the aftermath of the tragedy of September 11, the school killings of 2012, the Boston Marathon incident, and America's other similar violent acts, most U.S. families are re-examining their core values. Let's look at how we feed our children today. An overload of antibiotics and other toxic chemicals, GMO and GE in our produce and livestock, as well as more gluten and sugar in our processed foods, coincides with an alarming increase in the rate of childhood diseases such as diabetes, obesity, and cancer. The number of our children on medications for ADD, ADHD, autism, and Asperger's syndrome has skyrocketed. Experts warn that some of these medications often result in suicidal and violent tendencies, as well as chronic depression.

As a G-F–HSP, I am very frustrated about the lack of information the media provides about these threats to our children's mental and physical health. If we as individuals take responsibility for learning more about these issues without the media, perhaps our growing knowledge about the danger of these challenges plus the GMO threat, the lack of accurate food product labels, toxic food product packaging, and the increase of environmental toxins will spur parents and the rest of us to realize that unhealthy foods and the desire for convenience place a terrible burden of poor health on our planet's next generation.

What type of adults do we want to populate our planet in the near future? We need the next generation to be healthy, clear-thinking individuals who will redesign our planet into safe place on which to live. As a G-F–HSP, my vision for future child-bearing adults is to focus on and incorporate quality nutritional education and control from your first thought of adding a child to your life — before conception, during pregnancy, while breastfeeding, and in the food choices you make for your children as they mature and grow.

THE FAMILY MEAL AND YOUR FAMILY'S HEALTH

Did you know something as simple as family dinners can actually improve your own and your family's health and halt or prevent disease? CNN Health reported in that a recent study in the journal Pediatrics, showed that children who eat dinner with their families at least three nights per week are at a reduced risk for obesity, eating disorders, and they eat fewer unhealthy foods. This promising study shows that our kids' bodies do pay attention to what they eat; so the earlier we are able to introduce nutrient-dense foods, which include wild salmon, pasture-raised, soy-free chicken and eggs, grass-fed red meat, and raw, organic butter and other raw dairy products, the more they will pay attention and choose those foods on their own. The Weston A. Price Foundation website (*Westonprice.com*) has a full section on children's health, as well as a great post about packing the perfect lunchbox.

My son, Sacha, is now almost fifty years old. He was born in Rome in 1966. As we lived in Italy, the only English-speaking parenting book I could find was my mother's parenting bible, Dr. Spock from 25 years past. Massimo, my Florentine husband and Sacha's father, ridiculed me for turning to a book and not using my motherly instincts, which he believed all women should have. He thought I wasn't a natural mother, but I trusted Dr. Spock's common sense advice. I had no other American mothers to turn to in Rome, and at the time long distance telephone calls to Colorado were too expensive for anything but emergencies. I stopped nursing Sacha at five months and put him on solids, including semolina wheat.

Because there were no supermarkets in Rome in 1966, I spent most of my day in my little neighborhood shops as I marketed twice daily (Massimo wanted fresh rolls and bread from the baker), and then went home to prep and puree fruits and veggies, chop liver, cook chicken, beef, and grains so that he would have a choice of at least four items to choose from at each meal. He followed the Italian cultural mealtime ritual: The family eats together. Italian children taste a bit of everything their parents eat both at meals and snack time from the time they are infants, sometimes along with a tiny sip of good table wine to wash it down.

Italian babies eat homemade baby food until they graduate to finger food, and they devour spaghetti with their fingers until they can manage a fork. I loved to watch Bianca, my two-year-old granddaughter, wolf down her pasta with two fists at a time just as her papa did when he was a baby her age in Rome! It is rare to see an Italian child refuse food or act out in restaurants. No temper tantrums about food anywhere as a rule because food is a natural part of the Italian day's enjoyment. Everyone shares stories about the day's events at lunch and especially at the dinner table. Italians have begun to take a shorter lunch hour, eat fast food, and skip their naps. It will be interesting to see how the "American Way" influences their health.

Burgers and junk food were not yet part of the Italian food culture in 1966, although there was a Kentucky Fried Chicken on the Apian Way. Italians and the rest of the world are now hooked on junk food. Today, American wheat, which contributes to the majority of junk food today, is refused by most European and Asian nations. Asia is joining the bandwagon and refuses to buy US wheat until they can test it.

Reuters reported on 5/30/2013:

> "Japan has just cancelled a large contract to purchase U.S. wheat. 'We will refrain from buying western white and feed wheat effective today,' Toru Hisadome, a Japanese farm ministry official in charge of wheat trading.

> "As the USDA has admitted, experiments from 1998–2005 were held in open wheat fields. The genetically engineered wheat escaped and found its way into commercial wheat fields in Oregon (and possibly 15 other states) causing self-replicating genetic pollution that now affects the entire U.S. farmers' open field wheat industry.

> "South Korea, China, and the Philippines are waiting for the USDA to develop a testing kit, which is not in the works as yet."

> *http://www.reuters.com/article/2013/05/30*
> */us-wheat-asia-idUSL3N0EB1JC20130530*

Sacha and I only ate ice cream and dessert in the piazza when we went for an occasional walk after dinner. At home, dessert was fruit and cheese. Our only doctor was homeopathic, whom we visited occasionally for Sacha's tendency to get bronchitis (his father and I both smoked when I was pregnant and during his early childhood). While I was a macrobiotic for four years, I shopped for and cooked six different meals a day (three different dishes each at lunch and dinner) not counting extra dishes two to three times a week, when we had dinner guests. There was an average of five hours a day domestic time between all this, plus cleanup times. It was a normal routine at the time for Italian mothers and wives to spend most of their lives shopping, cooking and cleaning up, as most Italian women didn't work away from home at that time.

Cultural habits have since changed, and I look forward to seeing how the challenges working mothers pan out now that they don't have as much domestic support from their own parents and family.

Pamela Druckerman is an American who has lived in France for many years and raised her four children there. Her fun-to-read and valuable book, *Bringing Up Bebe*, shocks me with statistics that show France is number one in good health, and America rates at thirty-seven!

Her book also explains why French babies don't have the same eating behavioral problems that many American children have, because French babies have a combination of structure and freedom from the time they are born. If they act out, it is at home, never in restaurants. Their parents wouldn't allow it. In Italy, American children are known as intrusive and badly behaved. I never saw Italian children act out in restaurants with screams and rebellious behavior.

A new study, published in *JAMA Pediatrics*, aimed to estimate the economic impact of children's food allergies in the U.S. The researchers examined both the economic impacts and the willingness of caregivers to pay for treatment for food allergies. They examined a representative sample of caregivers for a child with a food allergy, looking at the period from November 28, 2011 to January 26, 2012.

Results of the study showed that the total national economic impact from children's food allergies was $24.8 billion or $4,184 per year per child with an allergy. Direct medical costs accounted for $4.3 billion annually, including emergency department visits, hospitalizations, and clinician visits. For the families of children with food allergies, the annual cost was $20.5 billion. This amount includes time off for medical visits, out-of-pocket medical costs, lost productivity, and opportunity costs. As a whole, caregivers were willing to pay more than the amount borne by families in total.

Medscape describes food allergies as "immunologically mediated adverse reactions to foods." A child or adult may suffer from an acute onset of symptoms following ingestion of the triggering food allergen, or a person may develop and suffer from a chronic disorder. Some of the symptoms of food allergies that have been observed in clinical settings are food-induced anaphylactic reactions that may involve the skin, gastrointestinal tract, and respiratory tract.

While it is possible for any food protein to trigger an allergic reaction, and a large number of foods have been documented as being clinical allergens, the majority of reactions can be accounted for with a small group of foods. Some of the more common food allergies confirmed in clinical settings are eggs, milk, peanuts, soy, fish, shellfish, tree nuts, wheat and strawberries. The confirmation of these allergens occurred through well-controlled, blinded food challenges that are medically supervised. In addition to these common allergens, sesame appears to be an emerging allergen.

According to an earlier National Monitor article, food allergies are increasingly common in the U.S. Currently, an estimated four to six percent of children are suffering from allergies. Food allergen exposure is also responsible for an estimated 300,000 emergency room visits for children. A severe response to allergens, known as anaphylaxis, has a 30% fatality rate. Scientists have also discovered that food allergies are not always permanent. For example, as many as 20% of people stop having peanut allergies as they get older. Gluten sensitivity may be permanent as it is usually hereditary and genetic.

WHAT ABOUT FISH? FRANKENFISH!

I will share more shocking information here, similar to what I have discussed about red meat in Chapter Five. My research about transgenics always shocks me. I feel that so much in the food industry goes on behind my back! A 2011 report from *The Independent Magazine* gives us the history of transgenic modification in the animal world—a science-fiction horror story we live each day when we go to grocery shop in our supermarkets.

The media doesn't share this detailed information about corporate extrinsic food industrialization. I find it in the medical journals I have permission to access and online research I do on a daily basis. Most families don't take time for in-depth research and depend on what their friends, family, and Dr. Oz tells them.

As the Organic Consumers Association (*www.organicconsumer.org*) writes about Frankenfish on its website in December, 2012:

> The first genetically engineered salmon—dubbed "Frankenfish"—could be in grocery stores and restaurants as early as 2014. The FDA is expected to approve AquaBounty Technologies' GE salmon after a 60-day public comment period. If approved, it will be the first approved food from a transgenic animal application to enter the U.S. food supply.
>
> Consumer and environmental activists oppose genetically engineered "Frankenfish" for many reasons, including the potential danger it poses to human health, to the environment and to the U.S. fishing economy.
>
> ### WHAT IS FRANKENFISH?
>
> AquaBounty Technologies, a Massachusetts-based biotech company, created the "AquAdvantage" salmon by injecting a fragment of DNA from an Ocean Pout fish, which is a type of eel, along with a growth hormone

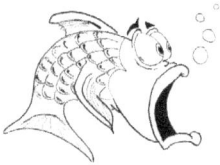

OPENING PANDORA'S BOX

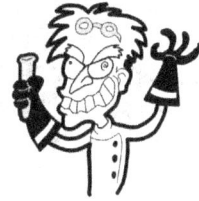

1980
Laboratory mice with genes inserted from other individuals become the first genetically modified "transgenic" animals. Dozens of other experimental species, from pigs and chickens to frogs and fish, follow over the next two decades.

1989
Microinjecting a fragment of DNA from an ocean pout fish and a Chinook Pacific salmon into a fertilized Atlantic creates The AquAdvantage founder salmon.

1995
AquaBounty Technologies begins the lengthy process of applying for official U.S. Government approval to develop the AquAdvantage salmon commercially.

2002
The first commercially viable GM animal is created from two species by Nexia Biotechnologies in rural Quebec. The "spider-goat" has a single gene from a golden orb-weaving spider which means its milk contains spiders silk, five times the strength of steel, which is used for making bulletproof vests.

2009
The U.S. Food and Drug Administration issues its final guidance to the GM industry on rules governing the regulation of genetically engineered animals, which clarifies its status as the chief statutory and regulatory body for GM animals.

2011
British scientists create chickens which don't spread bird flu by inserting an artificial gene that introduces a small part of the flu virus into the bird. This gives them the virus, but prevents them from spreading it.

2012
A genetically modified cow in New Zealand is the first to produce milk with no Beta-lacto globulin (BLG), the protein that is thought to be responsible for allergic reactions. Meanwhile, Chinese scientists create a GM cow whose milk includes Omega-3 fats, normally found in fish.

gene from the Chinook Pacific Salmon, into a fertilized Atlantic salmon egg. The result? A salmon that produces growth hormone year round, instead of only during warm weather. This allows the fish to reach market weight in just 18 months, instead of the usual three years.

WHAT ARE THE RISKS?

1. Potential harm to human health. The FDA has allowed this fish to move forward based on tests of allergenicity of only six GE fish. Even with such limited testing, the results showed an increase in allergy causing potential, according to Hansen. AquAdvantage also contains elevated levels of the growth hormone, IGF-1, which is linked to prostate, breast and colon cancers.

2. Potential harm to wild salmon population. Only 95% of the AquAdvantage salmon may be sterile, the rest fertile. Plus, the fish at the egg production facility in Prince Edward Island, Canada, will not be sterile. The FDA says the likelihood of the GE salmon escaping into the wild is "extremely remote" but gave little reassuring evidence to support that assumption. According to studies, the Frankenfish eat five times more food than wild salmon, and have less fear of predators. All it would take is for some of these Frankenfish to escape, and the world's wild salmon population would be at risk.

3. Frankenfish will be unlabeled. Without GMO labeling, consumers will not be able to avoid Frankenfish when it arrrives in grocery stores and fish markets.

http://salsa3.salsalabs.com/o/50865/p/dia/action3/common/public/?action_KEY=9142

These are only a few of the risks from genetic modification. My own research suggests that it is too late, and all but the tiny fish such as wild sardines are toxic. The FDA will have to listen when enough consumers demand that it adopt more reliable safety and testing measures for all its GMO products. Countries in Western Europe, Asia and India, prohibit GMO and no longer buy corn and soy from the U.S. because they are toxic.

The spectre of Frankenfood is one of the main issues that prompted me to create **The Family Meal**™ program in 2005. I wanted to find a fast-food restaurant sponsor who needed some good press and persuade them to incorporate a grass roots movement to incorporate a family meal in their customers' lives. Once a week, their customers with children could cook a healthy meal in their home where everyone cooks together and comes to the table to eat at the same time. The next step would be to invite the family of a neighbor family to share the whole experience, then a teacher from the child's school. The Family Meal could from there extend to the neighborhood, the community, and eventually the entire USA.

I targeted a fast-food restaurant such as McDonald's that serves what they call "healthy" foods and are already somewhat aware of how children are future customers. They now market to children and families with an on-the-premises playground, collectible toys and paper crowns. Wendy's even offers "gluten-free" food. I cover the gluten challenge in another chapter. The fast-food restaurant sponsor would provide free educational materials about healthy diets: CDs with simple recipes for gluten-free and fermented foods, entertaining cooking lesson videos, a food-related comic book, activities, and special bonuses. The program could be incorporated in the schoolroom as part of the curriculum.

As an example of this program, in 2008 I visited Alice Waters of Chez Panisse at her organic vegetable garden classroom at Martin Luther King Elementary School. The children were happily cooking the vegetables they had planted under the supervision of parent volunteers and teachers. All the children who participated in that part of the curriculum would enjoy the food they grew and prepared together at the school table, and then take the recipes to make the dishes at home with their families.

Barbara Kingsolver in her book *Animal, Vegetable, Miracle* writes that when she lived in New York and had a tiny vegetable garden she tried to teach the neighborhood children about gardening. Some of them didn't know that carrots grew in dirt and didn't want to touch the earth because it was dirty. She talks about how children today think vegetables come in plastic wrappings and only the wealthier people can afford to feed their families organic food.

This is something we can change easily, along with a gluten-free way of eating. Let's get together and enlist the media to publish more information on how to eat a truly healthy diet. Then we can teach the government how to eat and create a useful and accurate good pyramid, instead of our present one which focuses on grains and unhealthy products such as GMO corn and soy. Of course, the government wants us to eat more corn and soy because they have a surplus sitting in warehouses that no other country wants to buy from us.

Glutamine 1000mg gel caps under the tongue work well to counteract cravings as you adapt to doing without sugar and carbs. These cravings actually affect your brain as heroin does and result in foggy thinking, headaches, mood swings, and more cravings.

Gluten Society expert Dr. Peter Osborne, in the November 2, 2011 issue of his newsletter (*www.glutensociety.com*), offers valuable, free guidelines about how to avoid gluten:

Avoiding Gluten (Unsafe Ingredients for Gluten Sensitivity)

The following is a comprehensive (but not complete) list of foods that do contain gluten or that may contain it. This list can be used as a guideline for those with gluten intolerance or celiac disease. Many items listed below are traditionally considered safe. It should be noted, however, that many of the traditionally safe grains have been studied to cause and to contribute to damage yet they continue to be recommended by the corporate gluten-free food industry. The difference between a traditional gluten-free diet and the TRUE gluten free diet can be found in the following video tutorial:

http://www.glutenfreesociety.org/video-tutorial/gluten-sensitivity-what-is-it/

TRUE Gluten-Free Diet Guidelines
Avoid All of These...

· Amaranth***
· Barley (malt)
· Buckwheat***
· Corn (maize)*
· Durum (semolina)
· Einkorn****
· Emmer
· Graham
· Groat
· Millet*
· Oats
· Quinoa***
· Rice* (does not include wild rice varieties but does include brown rice)

· Rye
· Sorghum*
· Spelt*
· Teff*
· Triticale
· Wheat****

*These grains are classically considered gluten free, but are not recommended on a TRUE gluten free diet as they are classified as cross-grains due to genetic modification and chemicals in the soil.

***These items are technically not grains, but are at high risk for cross-contamination and not recommended on a TRUE gluten-free diet unless verification can be obtained. These pseudo cereals are also very high in glutamic acid and should be discouraged as substitutes for patients with neurological symptoms.

****Note: there is no such thing as a complete comprehensive list of food items that contain gluten. Manufacturers regularly change their ingredients, mislabel, have product recalls, etc. This is why Gluten Free Society's stance is to avoid processed and packaged foods as much as possible, as well as to avoid eating out as much as possible."

At Young Living Essential Oil's annual convention in 2013, Dr. Schreuder, Young Living's research scientist (*www.youngliving.com*) suggests exchanging *all* grains for greens in your diet. YLEO is currently growing Einkorn wheat, the planet's first wheat, with only 14 chromosomes. Our current durum wheat has 42 and is very hard to digest. It will apparently be good for those with CD and gluten intolerance. The Italians are also researching a wheat species that allows more gluten tolerance for a culture whose food is based on wheat.

After I dropped all grain products, my focus and stamina increased considerably. Dr. Schreuder says dropping *all* grains will decrease inflammation in the body. He says to avoid roots and focus more on nuts. The more grains we eat, he says, the faster our brains decline!

Mike Adams, owner of the Gluten-Free Society, has a valuable newsletter and offers the following tips:

Misc. Food Additives or Processed Foods That Can Contain Gluten

- Agave Syrup — High in sugar
- Artificial Colors
- Artificial Flavors
- Bouillon cubes or stock cubes
- Candy may be dusted with wheat flour; ask.
- Canned soups — Most are not acceptable.
- Caramel color and flavoring
- Cheese spreads & other processed cheese foods.
- Chocolate — May contain malt flavoring.
- Cold cuts, Wieners, Sausages — May have gluten due to cereal fillers.
- Dextrin
- Dip mixes
- Dry sauce mixes
- Extenders and binders
- Honey, except organic raw
- Honey Hams — Can be based with wheat starch in coating.
- Hydrogenated Starch Hydrolysate
- Hydrolyzed plant protein
- Hydrolyzed vegetable protein
- Hydroxypropylated Starch
- Ice Cream & Frozen Yogurt — Check all dairy for casein.
  Cows are fed grains and many react to dairy for this reason.
  Grass fed, raw dairy recommended (or avoid dairy altogether).
- Instant Teas & Coffees — Cereal products may be included in the formulation.
- Maltodextrin (wheat or corn based)

· Maltose
· Mayonnaise — Check thickener and grain based vinegar ingredients
· Modified food starch (I buy Follow Your Heart's soy-free Veganaise.)
· MSG
· Mustard — Mustard powder may contain gluten
· Natural Colors
· Natural Flavors
· Non Dairy Creamer
· Oil, frying — Check for cross-contamination or corn-based oils.
· Pregelatinized starch
· Seasonings — Check labels
· Smoke flavors
· Soy Miso
· Soy Sauce
· Textured vegetable protein
· Vegetable gum
· Vegetable protein
· Baking powder — Commonly contains grain – wheat or corn
· Dry roasted nuts & honey roasted nuts
· French fries in restaurants — Same oil may be used for wheat-containing items.
· Gravies — Check out thickening agent and liquid base.
· Poultry and meats — Check out flavorings & basting, inquire about meat glue
· Sour cream — May contain modified food starch of indeterminate source.
· Vitamin supplements — Check the labels carefully; different brands contain grain-based ingredients

The Grasses — Many people want to use wheat, barley, rye, and oat grass (not the seed) as a supplement in the gluten-free diet. Technically, these do not contain gluten, as they are the grass part of the plant. However, it is recommended that these be avoided to prevent the possibility of cross contamination.

Alcoholic Beverages That Contain Gluten

· Beer (G-F beer is not gluten-free as it is made from a grain)
· Grain based spirits — Many claim that distillation removes gluten; Gluten-Free Society recommends avoidance regardless
· Malted beverages

Vodka and Tequila are permissible on occasion as they are not grain- or cross-grain based; however, they convert to sugar and affect the immune system. They can also cause inflammation.

Non Edible Items That May Contain Gluten (Read Your Labels)

· Crayons
· Detergents
· Hairspray & Shampoo
· Lipstick
· Lotions
· Makeup
· Medications & Vitamins
· Pet Food
· Play-Doh
· Stamps & envelopes
· Toothpaste

SOURCE: *www.theglutenfreesociety.com*

I want you to be sure to leave extra time when grocery shopping. Offer your young children a healthy treat at the end if they cooperate when you take the extra time to read labels. When you do buy packaged foods, be sure to take time read the label carefully. There are popular movements online and locally to buy local organic and support the farmers markets, which is my first choice when I market. Google it!

A PARTIAL LIST OF HEALTHY, GLUTEN-FREE FOODS AND BEVERAGES.

Buy local and organic whenever possible and check the labels
and manufacturers to see if they are produced in
a non-contaminated farm, kitchen, or factory:

Avocados

Bananas

Chia Seeds

Chickpea (Garbanzo Bean) Miso

Cider Vinegar

Coconut Butter

Coconut Cream

Coconut Kefir (easy to make)

Coconut Mana

Coconut Milk (best fresh)

Coffee

Chicken Broth In between Meals

Grapeseed Oil

Grass-fed organic chickens

Grass-fed, organic, non-GMO
    red meat

Kelp Pasta

Kombucha (easy to make)

Nut Butters (organic)

Olive Oil

Perpetual Bone Soup

Pineapple

Raw Cacao Powder

Raw Milk Cheeses (especially goat
    cheese, from grass-fed milk)

Raw, Soaked Nuts

Raw, Soaked Seeds

Sea Veggies

Slice of lemon, mint, and/or
    cucumber in cool water

Soy-free egg yolks
    (whites are often allergenic)

Sugarless Dark Chocolate

Tamari (wheat-free)

Tea

Tequila

Vegetables (organic, non-GMO)

Vodka

Wild Berries

Wild Salmon

WHAT NOW?

MY GLUTEN-FREE REGIME

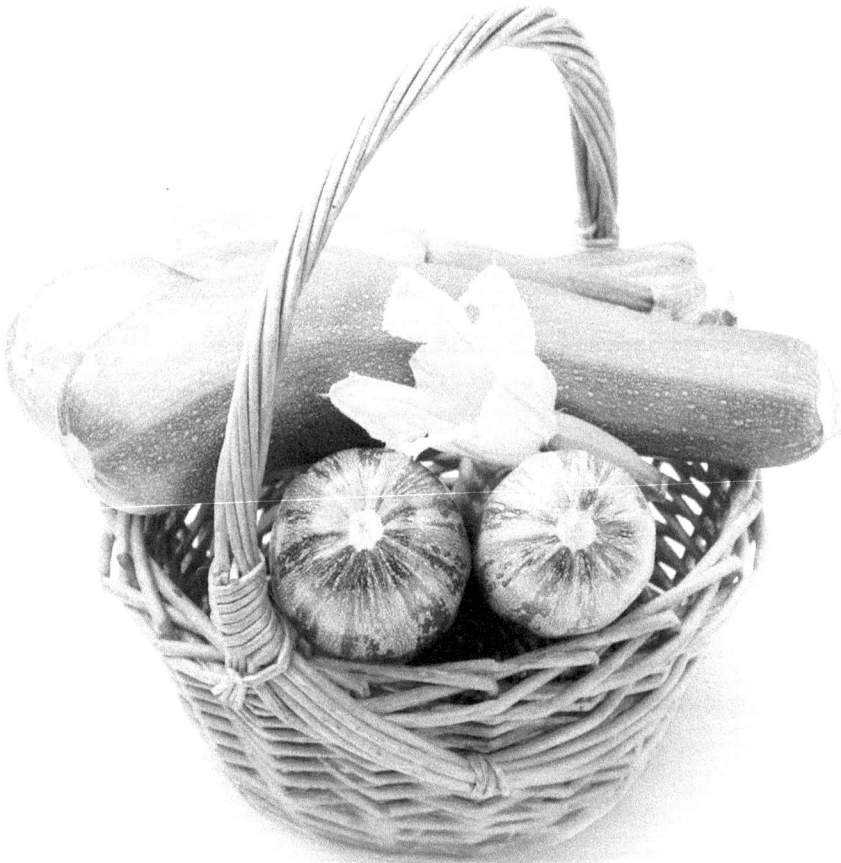

Ancora Primo

These tasty little fritters are very convenient for summer meals and last-minute gatherings. You can bake them instead of frying. They are delicious at room temperature and also freeze well. Wrap two in parchment paper and you can take them out whenever you need them.

Gluten-Free Zucchini Fritters with Herb Vinaigrette

SERVES 6

INGREDIENTS

Vinaigrette

1 cup soy-free veganaise or other gluten-free mayonnaise
¼ cup fresh dill, chopped
¼ cup fresh chives, chopped
2 Tbsp. fresh tarragon, chopped
2 Tbsp. fresh Italian parsley, chopped
1 Tbsp. apple cider vinegar
1 Tbsp. salted capers, soaked
1 anchovy fillet, chopped
½ cup grapeseed or coconut oil

Fritters — Makes 12 fritters

1½ pounds medium zucchini (5 to 6), trimmed
1½ teaspoons coarse quality salt, divided
6½ Tbsp. coconut flour
½ teaspoon baking powder
½ teaspoon freshly ground black pepper
¼ cup purified water
1 4-ounce package soft, fresh goat cheese, coarsely crumbled, chilled
    (about 1 cup)
⅓ cup (or more) extra-virgin olive oil
3½ cups (lightly packed) mâche (lamb's lettuce) or arugla

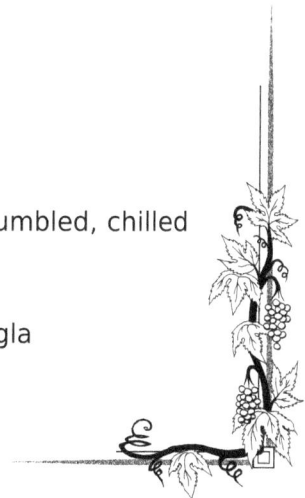

PREPARATION

VINAIGRETTE

Blend all ingredients in processor until smooth, occasionally scraping down sides of bowl. Season dressing with salt and pepper.

Transfer to small bowl. Cover; chill.

Can be made 1 day ahead. Keep chilled.

FRITTERS

Using large holes on box grater, coarsely grate zucchini into large colander. Sprinkle 1 teaspoon coarse salt over and toss to coat evenly. Place colander over large bowl. Let zucchini stand 30 minutes, tossing occasionally.

Press on zucchini to release as much liquid as possible. Empty zucchini into kitchen towel. Roll up to enclose and squeeze dry.

Whisk flour, baking powder, ½ teaspoon pepper, and ½ teaspoon coarse salt in medium bowl to blend. Mix in beer.

Scrape zucchini from towel into bowl; stir to coat evenly (batter will be thick). Mix in cheese.

Heat ⅓ cup oil in heavy large skillet over medium heat until very hot, about 2 minutes.

Working in batches, drop batter into skillet by ¼ cupfuls, flattening to 3-inch rounds. Sauté until brown and cooked through, 4 to 5 minutes per side.

Transfer fritters to rimmed baking sheet. Repeat with remaining batter, adding more oil as needed. DO AHEAD: Can be made 2 hours ahead. Let stand at room temperature. Rewarm in 375°F oven 5 to 6 minutes.

Place mâche or arugula in large bowl. Toss with 2 to 3 tablespoons dressing. Place 2 fritters on each of 6 plates. Top with mound of mâche salad.

Serve fritters, passing remaining dressing alongside.

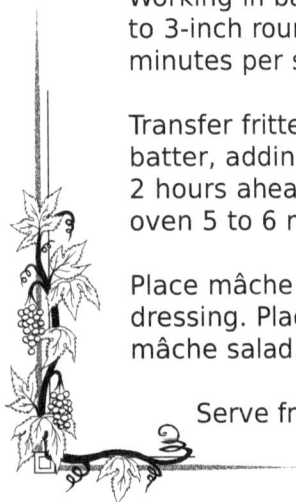

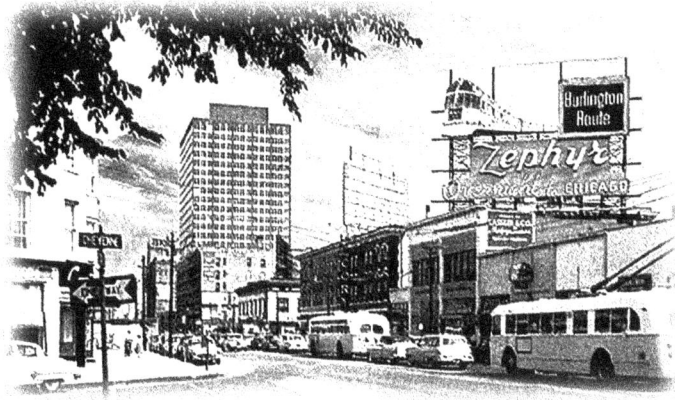

hen I grew up with "real" food in a very fifties culture in Middle America, Denver, Colorado, I didn't know that agricultural techniques such as extrinsic food production existed to "enhance" my food's appearance, or that processed foods are toxic and diminish taste. As I developed my palate in my late teens and traveled to Europe, I enjoyed food from many European countries that tasted more delicious because they were authentic and unadulterated.

Now, most of the food I eat here in the U.S. is adulterated with chemicals: sprayed, dipped, radiated, and genetically modified (GMO). As consumers become more informed and demand cleaner and tastier food, I find more "natural" and local pasture-raised, grass-fed, and organic foods to choose from here in California. I still have to deal, however, with the FDA's recommendations and lack of precise labeling. I don't trust the manufacturers or the health food markets unless I research the food manufacturers themselves when I buy processed and packaged foods that claim to be "free" of gluten and chemicals. I do trust the organic farmers I have gotten to know at the farmers markets.

Many people lose or gain weight in the first month of the gluten-free diet, and experience fewer migraines, joint aches, digestive problems, depression, and other gluten sensitivity symptoms. Because we are all very unique physically, mentally, and spiritually, I feel we must be responsible to do our individual, independent research to find the ideal solution to each of our own personal dietary challenges.

This G-F diet takes patience, energy, and time. I am learning to make myself slow down and notice how I feel after I eat, take time to read labels in detail when I market, search out and support local farmers markets, refuse toxic food product packaging.

When my MD, who is also an alternative healer, diagnosed me with gluten intolerance, she told me that I should eliminate *all* grains because I had *dysbiosis* (an allergy to grains and their cross-links) because of disaccharides. Dysbiosis (also called dysbacteriosis) is a theory of having microbial imbalances on or within the body. Dysbiosis is most prominent in the digestive tract or on the skin, but can also occur on any exposed surface or mucous membrane such as the vagina, lungs, nose, sinuses, ears, nails or eyes. These molecules contribute to gluten intolerance because they cause more inflammation for the immune system. This results in autoimmune disease, which limits our ability to absorb the nutrients we need to prevent disease. I do feel better much better without grains and high carb veggies such as potatoes and acorn squash in my diet, though I eat them on occasion.

MY PALEO DIET AND A SAMPLE MENU:

I don't recommend my personalized diet to anyone other than my clients, as each of us must design our own plan according to our individual needs. In Chapter Five I give a brief discussion about the issues of vegetarianism and extrinsic food production, and discuss some ideas and biases about whether "To Meat or Not To Meat." In the meantime, I eat a basic Paleo-style menu three meals a day and a couple of snacks that include one of the following at least once a week: raw grass-fed beef, organic liver, organic bacon, some cooked organic free-range soy-free fowl and eggs, game, wild mercury-free fish and seafood, organic berries, organic Granny Smith apples, some sea vegetables, and organic, raw, soaked nuts and seeds.

I use a handful or two of Lacinato (Dino) Italian kale at most meals. I steam the kale so it is always ready to eat with other dishes, and sometimes eat it raw in salads. I do better with cooked vegetables than with raw foods and salads. I don't eat grains or cross-grains, except for one of the following on occasion: a brown rice tortilla or Asian rice paper wraps.

My Typical G-F Menu for the Day

Breakfast 3 Egg yolks and 1 white (cooked soft, fried, poached, or scrambled), sautéed kale, 2 small strips organic bacon, herbal tea or warm coconut milk with raw carob powder, or coconut kefir, organic carrot juice, grass-fed lamb chop, or wild salmon. (I am allergic to egg whites, as are many people with gluten sensitivity and other allergies.)

Lunch Sautéed or poached wild salmon or pastured chicken, buffalo burger, steamed arugula, kale, escarole, endive, watercress, fresh herbs goat cheese wild sardines or wild smoked salmon.

Snack Granny Smith apple.

Dinner Ground turkey or ground buffalo as meatballs or meatloaf, with raw, organic, homemade ketchup, lamb sirloin steak, buffalo Clod roast cut sliced very thin and sautéed, organic pastured chicken, kale, and stir-fried or steamed broccoli, dandelion, asparagus or other steamed greens.

Snack Veggies and protein or nuts.

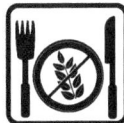

My favorite dessert of the moment is raw honey, organic carob powder (from Nativas, my favorite super food company, coconut manna or oil, and fresh or frozen wild, organic raspberries sweetened with stevia. This makes a truffle. I use a product named Xylitol that is one-for one with sugar. It is better to use organic coconut sugar if you don't like Xylitol.

I don't do a lot of baking, because of the cross-grains, but once in awhile I bake a gluten-free banana bread to eat with organic lemon curd made with soy-free eggs. For sweeteners, I use Xylitol as a sugar substitute. Agave syrup is highly processed and full of fructose.

Now that I have taken the time to do the work to understand my body and emotions better, I upgrade my regime daily according to my instinct. Since I became gluten-free, I start my day with a ritual of spiritual reading, prayers, breathing and yoga, I am more in touch with myself now. I ask myself what I want to eat when I get up in the morning and throughout the day, and shop once a week so I will have a good choice of healthy foods on hand. Sometimes I prepare more to freeze or for a special treat or gift for friends and clients.

I am very fortunate because I love to menu plan, market, cook, and eat. I know many people would rather get takeout or eat in restaurants because they don't like to have to think about it and are too busy and stressed to have one more thing to worry about in their hectic lives. These people see food as just one more problem. That's one of the main reasons I wrote this book. I want to encourage people to take responsibility for themselves and our children to create a healthier and more joyous planet through a healthful attitude and food practice. I also surround myself with people who do EAT REAL so my three-year-old grand daughter and I enjoy our lives with like-minded people.

Sometimes, I prepare food in the morning for the rest of the day so I save time for coaching sessions, writing, research, and socializing later in the day. I am very pleased with the results of my mindful attitude about my daily regime—I have more energy, more stable emotions, no tummy aches, (unless I cheat), no depression, and increased brain clarity. When I fall off this regime because I have an emotional upset or get bored, I revert to Donna Gates *Body Ecology Program (the B.E.D.)*, which fits my regime and is a change of pace from my daily routine.

We are what we eat and so much more. Our food choices and habits are reflected in our thoughts and feelings about our planet's environment, our societal and political issues, and our connection (or lack of connection) to "Something Greater Than Ourselves." The statistics that Lisa Miller stated in her *Newsweek* article are alarming: "More than one-third of U.S. adults and 17 percent of children are obese, and the problem is acute among the poor." And other sources indicate that these numbers are rising at an alarming rate Childhood diabetes is a new threat.

The effects of gluten on the body and mind have similar consequences when carbohydrates from grains, starchy vegetables, and most fruits convert to sugar and create what is called the *metabolic syndrome* —uncontrollable cravings that can become addictions that alter the brain, body, and emotions.

In a similar manner, people who are alcoholics, drug abusers, and smokers often develop wheat and sugar addictions because they have a genetic disposition to the sugar in carbohydrates. Men especially crave sugar to repress their anxious thoughts and women want sugar, especially chocolate, to quiet their stressful feelings. Sugar can create an endless cycle of cravings and mood swings that lead to over-secretion of *cortisol*, a brain hormone that can lead to life threatening diseases that are caused by the sugar and other drugs we use to relieve stress. Sugar's chemical effect on the brain is similar to that of heroin.

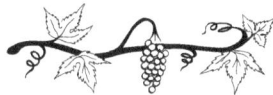

I remember after I first met Massimo, and I was living and working in Manhattan in an exclusive art gallery on Madison Avenue one block from Fifth Avenue. Massimo taught me how to cook in my fifth-floor walkup on the West Seventies, a block from Central Park. Italian men all know how to cook, even if they have never lifted a finger in the kitchen. They learn by osmosis as they watch their mothers. Massimo wanted me to cook like his mother, and tricked me by having me cook the traditional holiday foods as if he had always eaten them on a daily basis growing up. I found out about this trick after I lived in Italy for a while. Massimo celebrated Christmas every day and I cooked my little heart out for him.

The first dish he taught me was zabaglione, a dish that is a classic recipe that is said to restore energy after physical exertion. We had it after making love, and when skiing. A favorite secret of Italian lovers and athletes is an egg and sugar based recipe that is bottled and enjoyed as "Vov." He wanted me to cook every Sunday for five of his Italian male friends and there was always a lot of food, wine, and laughter while I was in the kitchen. But no one helped clean up! The first dinner party recipe Massimo taught me to cook was the Tuscan version of minestrone, Rebollito, a Florentine classic made from minestrone leftovers and dried bread.

Tuscan minestrone requires a huge amount of chopping and is very laborious. The first time I made it, I was still living alone, while Massimo often spent the night. I had carried my shopping bags after work from several markets on Ninth Avenue taken the subway and dragged them up five flights of stairs to my one-bedroom apartment. I chopped for a couple of hours in my tiny, cluttered kitchen. Massimo came over and popped his head around the corner.

"What are you doing?" he demanded.
"Making minestrone!" I replied as I looked up from my cutting board.
"That is minestrone for cows," he sneered, "not for people!"

I was devastated. I burst into tears and ran into the other room sobbing. I eventually finished the minestrone, and his guests ate it without complaints. Massimo continued to be critical about my cooking for the twenty years we were together, with an occasional compliment to keep me in the kitchen. We had guests for dinner two or three times a week for twenty years, and I spent a minimum of five hours a day marketing, cooking, and cleaning up. When I became a Radical Feminist and a macrobiotic chef that changed radically, and is another story.

I eventually left Massimo and, twenty years later when he was dying of pancreatic cancer, I went to Rome and cooked lunch and dinner for him and his friends until he died. It was a feast and a party for several people every day. I made him all his favorite dishes. He was on morphine, but still had a few criticisms about my cooking, even though he mostly enjoyed his childhood comfort food. Tuscans and other Italians in general are so dependent on their mothers' cooking they literally can't live without it. It's their anchor to Life and they spend much of their life eating, discussing what they are eating, where they ate it last, where it tasted better, and where they are going to eat it next.

When I first moved to Italy, I thought this whole ritual was ridiculous and over the top, but now, when I see the opposite in the U.S., and the painful results of increased diseases and apathy to nutrition, I follow the Italian approach when I talk with my gluten-free friends about our food and restaurant preference. Italians love of food may seem extreme but as a culture they have closer family ties, more playful and spontaneous, less stress, and are more creative in the way they live their daily lives. Granted, they are more Americanized now, and come from thousands of years of a diverse cultural mix. Italians don't always go home for lunch and take long naps today, but they still go out for a walk and a treat after dinner with their family and friends, and drink their endless espressos and eat fanini in their favorite café during breaks from work or while marketing.

I want to share my daily regime so you can understand better about why I eat the way I do. I did a hair analysis recently, and my doctor gave me an entirely new diet. I was diagnosed as a Fast Metabolizer type. That means I am high energy but burn out faster than I should and am low on energy reserves, low on minerals, and high on heavy metals. I still have a lot to improve about my health and the gluten-free diet was just the beginning

I repeat — I am a fast-metabolism type as diagnosed by my doctor. I do not recommend this diet to anyone unless they find out what type of metabolizer they are.

Now I eat like an Italian and also a Health Foodie — healthy longevity, not just for the taste. My taste buds adjust as I invent new foods to cook the G-F translated Italian recipes I have used for 40 years. I remember when I tried to figure out how to deal with my dysfunctional marriage and how I dealt with those dietary challenges. I learned it's most important to have a strong intent or dream for whatever I took on in life, and that you stand for your values. Otherwise, it is very difficult to be consistent when you try to change your patterns that don't work well.

A Tavola
Mangiamo!

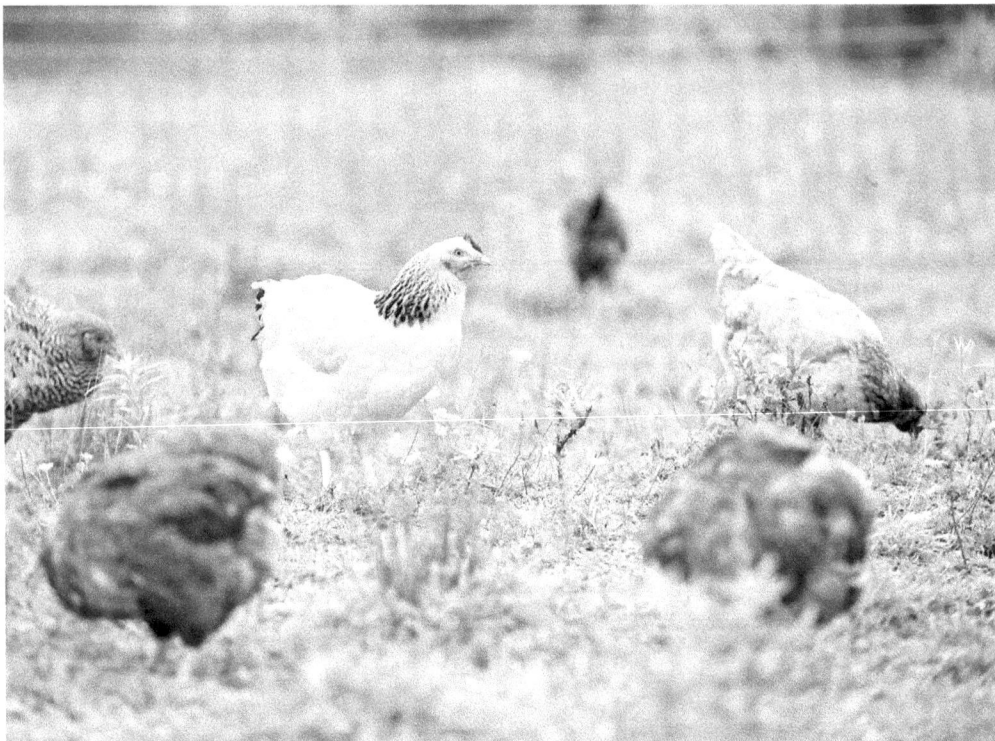

ANCORA! ANOTHER PRIMO PIATTO

This crispy and delectable chicken is one of the Sarchielli family's favorite recipes and also an excellent item for light lunches and picnics when served hot, cold, as a chicken salad, or at room temperature. It was a popular item at one of my favorite restaurants in Florence, Buca Del Orafo. Cook at a high heat on the grill or in a cast iron skillet on the stove.

CRISPY CHICKEN UNDER A BRICK

SERVES 6

INGREDIENTS

3½ pound organic, pastured chicken, backbone removed
1 Tbsp. quality salt plus more
½ teaspoon freshly ground black pepper plus more for seasoning
1 Tbsp. fresh organic rosemary or 1 teaspoon dried, minced
1 Tbsp. fresh, organic sage or q teaspoon dried, minced
1 Tbsp. organic olive oil
Special equipment: One brick, wrapped in foil, or a large cast-iron skillet.

PREPARATION

Open chicken and place on a work surface, skin side up. Using your palms, firmly press on breastbone to flatten the breast. Season chicken all over with 1 tablespoon salt, lemon zest, the herbs, and pepper.

Place in a greased baking dish and rub with 1 tablespoon oil. Let stand at room temperature for 1 hour.

To Grill:
Build a medium-low fire in a charcoal grill, or heat a gas grill to medium.

Place chicken, skin side down, on grill and place a brick or heavy skillet on top of chicken to weigh it down. (This will expose more skin to direct heat, making it crispy; the chicken will also cook faster.)

Cook until skin is crispy and golden brown, about 15 minutes. Using tongs, set brick aside.

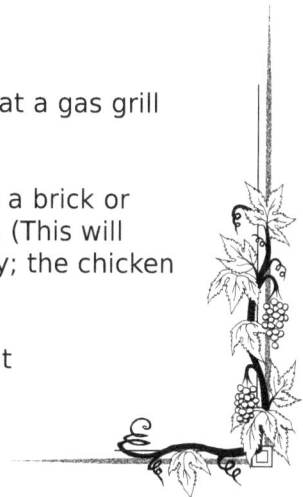

Turn chicken, cover grill, and cook for 10 more minutes. Continue cooking and turning chicken every 10 minutes, covering grill between turns, until an instant-read thermometer inserted into the thickest part of the thigh registers 165°F, about 50 minutes total.

Transfer to a carving board; let chicken rest for 10–20 minutes. (Resting will make for juicier meat.)

While chicken rests, add more coals to the fire if necessary to increase heat to medium, or heat gas grill to medium-high

Grill (or use a grill basket) over medium heat, turning occasionally, until softened and charred in spots, about 12 minutes.

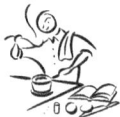

Chef's Note

Rub with 1/4-teaspoon cayenne pepper if you prefer it with a spicier flavor (al Diavolo).

Serve with red or white Chianti.

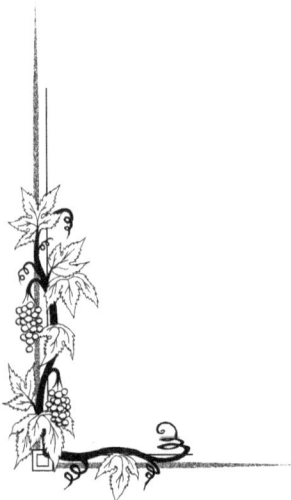

*A*fter I separated from Massimo in the early 1980s, I never returned to Rome until he was dying. Massimo stayed in Italy while I muddled through in Denver as a single mother. After I recuperated from cancer, I led a cooking tour to Siena in 1995 and taught cooking to a group of twelve students. After the lessons, on a visit to a friend in Milan, I was inspired by the Slow Food Movement and became a food activist focusing on social change through the food we grow and eat.

I returned to Denver after my cooking tour, opened a chapter of Slow Foods USA, and later opened two more chapters in Berkeley and San Francisco. I had also been working part-time as a temporary worker for international corporations in their marketing departments. I learned more about computers there under fire and went to computer school. My first full-time position in marketing was with The American Humane Association, which hired me as their PR Manager. I loved my job. After a year, however, I lost it to a space astronaut who had more political clout.

Over a period of ten years, from 1974 to 1984, I worked for Three Tomatoes Catering, which is still in business as I write. For twenty-five years, I also taught monthly Tuscan cuisine for the Denver Botanic Gardens and private students, I still had never heard of CD. My Tuscan pastas and lasagna recipes were my cooking students' and catering clients' favorites, and I continued to eat pasta and pizza when Sacha left for college. I continued to sell my accessory designs to boutiques and galleries in Denver, Aspen, Los Angeles and Taos, New Mexico.

I finally left belief in Massimo in the 1980s. It took almost twenty years to let go of my denial that we could heal our marriage. He had refused marriage counseling. I finally felt free! Sacha graduated from high school and was off to college on the East Coast with a partial scholarship, and my dog, Frisbee was my only responsibility.

After only four therapy sessions with EMDR (Emotional Disassociation Response), in 1996 I decided to move my caravan to the Bay Area. My Denver temp agency sent me on an assignment to IBM's international marketing department in San Francisco. I got a six-months sublet next door to my best friend of 29 years, and commuted every day on the BART. I had always loved San Francisco ever since my college days there as an art student.

And yet I kept dreaming about returning to Italy to live. While I was in California, I opened two Slow Food USA conviviums. Our convivium in Berkley was part of Alice Waters of Chez Panisse fame — the organic, locavore food pioneer.

I also taught cooking at Sur La Table stores in Berkeley and San Francisco, and in private homes. My IBM marketing assignment ended after six months, when they chose to give it to an IBM employee due to security risks with a temporary employee. Time to relocate my caravan again. I still had no inkling that I was gluten-sensitive, however, and I continued to have severe mood swings and anxiety, which topped my list of other disturbing symptoms.

Still gypsying my away around the world, in 1996 I was on my way back to Italy to live and stopped in Los Angeles to visit Sacha just days before the 9/11 Twin Towers disaster. After that, I didn't feel safe to travel and found a job as a kitchen designer, translator, and cooking instructor, for the French company, Demarle International. I designed their professional teaching kitchen and taught their sales force to use Demarle's high technology cooking tools. I also taught at Williams Sonoma and Sur la Table in Santa Monica.

In 1997, the Los Angeles Demarle office folded, and I was an unemployed celiac gypsy who had still not yet heard of gluten. I felt extremely anxious about my future, and my depression and mood swings became more severe.

I joined the Whole Foods Market team in the San Fernando Valley, where I created and developed their first cooking school. I expanded our customer base as I taught popular Tuscan cuisine classes for adults and children. Many of our customers had allergies to wheat. When doctors recommended wheat elimination to our Whole Foods customers, they grew confused and asked me, "What *can* I eat?"

This led to my creating a new position for myself as Whole Food's first food coach and gluten expert. I discovered through the intense research I did, to find solutions for my customers' nutrition, that I might be gluten intolerant. My research showed me that most wheat allergy symptoms are similar to those of gluten sensitivity and Celiac disease. I was grateful and compassionate for my customers and delved even deeper into the research. My customers' doctors had never mentioned gluten or CD. I suggested that Whole Foods buy some G-F products, but they laughed!

In 1997, 95% of celiacs were unaware that they had this potentially life-threatening disease. It took an average of 8 to 11 years and several thousands of dollars in doctors' visits and tests for an American celiac to be properly diagnosed. My own family doctor and homeopath confirmed my suspicions after I consulted with them. My homeopath suggested I might have Sjorgen's Disease, another label I had never heard of. This is a very scary journey I was on, and I was determined to solve the mystery of my symptoms and heal myself.

After I discovered the information about gluten, I began to eliminate anything suspicious from my diet. At this time, gluten was considered an intolerance or sensitivity, not an allergy. In 2011 we learned it can be all three. I had finally found the key to my continuous struggle for physical and mental balance. I had a gluten challenge! Maybe I am a Celiac!

I was both relieved to discover why I have suffered for all these years and frightened about the consequences. I asked myself if I, a chef whose world as an HSP food gypsy is defined through food and who lives to eat delicious and unique foods on a daily basis and share feast-like meals with my friends, have to deny myself my favorite foods? How will I enjoy my food if I have to do without wheat, barley, and rye? Will the cancer return? I didn't know at this time that gluten elimination is only the first step in a gluten-free regime.

In 1994, I had a mastectomy, chemo, radiation, and Tamoxifin for breast cancer and almost died from a rare staph infection. Afterwards, I revised my diet to include more dark green vegetables and less red meat (I am an O blood type and need a good amount of animal protein). I didn't do well as a vegetarian, and I was allergic to soy. Soy is toxic for many people as most of it is genetically modified and hard to digest unless fermented. It is also one of the top allergens. Cancer forced me into a harsh reality when I saw how depression, anger, and repression had contributed to this disease that almost took my life. I took Chinese herbs and had acupuncture, and maintained a grateful and positive attitude while I was healing. Cancer had turned my life around. I was ready to start my life over with a more positive attitude and a powerful intent to be as healthy as possible for the rest of my life.

In 2011, I went to Rome to help Massimo through the last stages of pancreatic cancer. I marketed and cooked meals three times a day to entertain at least ten of his friends a day at his table with all his favorite pastas and pastries. It was too late for a gluten-free diet for him at that stage of his life. While in

Italy, I attempted to teach my own friends and family there about the dangers of gluten. Even though they were familiar with the gluten danger, they couldn't imagine going without their daily pasta, bread, and desserts. They were stunned by my suggestion that they reduce the amount of wheat in their diet, and a few laughed at the idea.

At a dinner party in Milan, my closest Italian friend reluctantly promised to cut down on the wheat, but everyone there looked at me as if I needed a psychiatrist. After all, Italy has one of the highest incidences of Celiac Disease on the planet. Italian food habits are cultural and deeply ingrained over thousands of years. They borrowed the original pizza recipe from the ancient Greeks and turned it into a favorite of children and adults worldwide. It will take a few generations for them to stop their denial and to understand the life-threatening consequences of wheat and gluten on their lives.

I am still working out my own version of my personal gluten-free diet as I continue to discover and test new ideas and products daily. This is a never-ending process because of my unique personality and challenges. I love this process because I learn to know myself better and handle my emotions and emotional reactions better. I feel more joyful than I ever imagined possible. Each individual must take responsibility and research the G-F issue. The most important thing is to get in touch with your feelings and instinct and slow down enough to learn to listen to and trust them and the experts.

I am grateful to my life coaches and therapists and am now able to pass all my life experience on as a marketing coach for creative entrepreneurs.

You will find more resources about the gluten challenge in the following chapters.

9

FAD OR FOLLY?

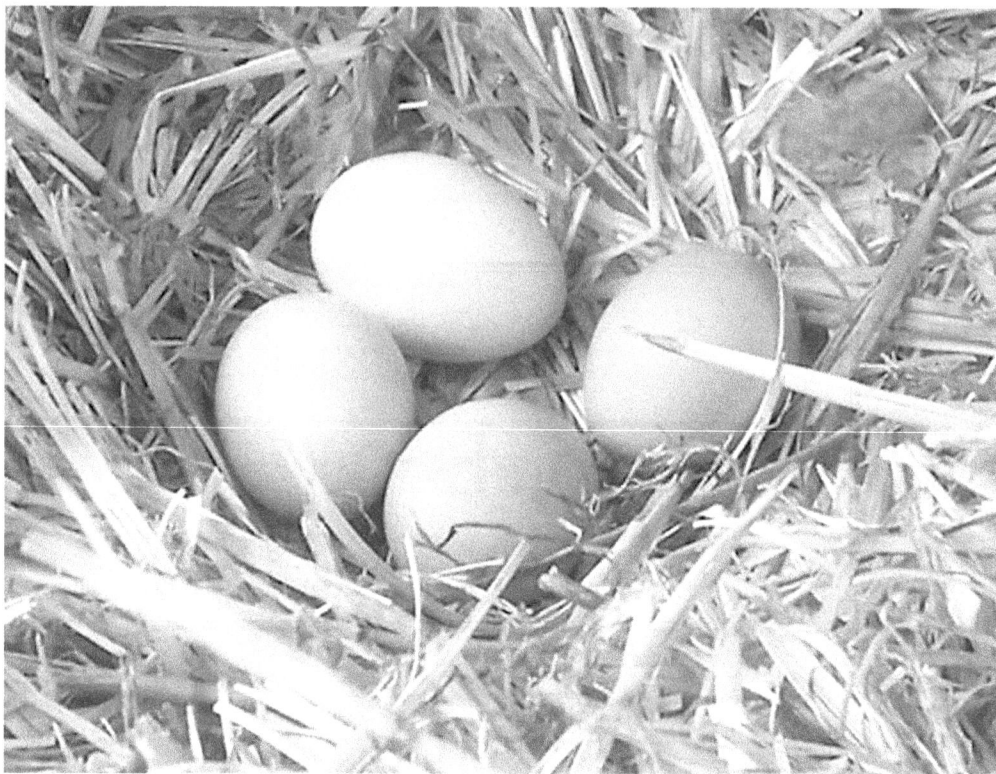

DOLCE (DESSERT)

Zabaglione is a traditional and delicious Italian dessert favored by lovers and athletics because it restores energy immediately after strenuous exercise. This recipe can be prepared in 45 minutes or less. Just enough time to take a breather!

ZABAGLIONE FOR GYPSY LOVERS

SERVES 2

INGREDIENTS

4 organic, soy-free, pastured, large egg yolks
¼ cup organic coconut sugar
½ cup dry Marsala

PREPARATION

Have an instant-read thermometer ready in a cup of hot water.
In a metal bowl with a whisk or a hand-held electric mixer, beat
together all ingredients until combined well.

Set bowl over a saucepan of barely simmering water and beat
mixture until tripled in volume and thermometer registers 140°F,
about 5 minutes.

To ensure that eggs are cooked, beat mixture 3 minutes more.

Put some on a tablespoon and run a finger through the mixture.
If it leaves a groove it is ready.

Serve zabaglione immediately.

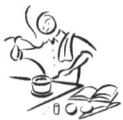

Chef's Note

Tempting alone, it's even better spooned over fresh or grilled fruit or served with gluten-free biscotti. Have whatever you plan to serve with the zabaglione ready to go. It is best-enjoyed seconds off the stove.

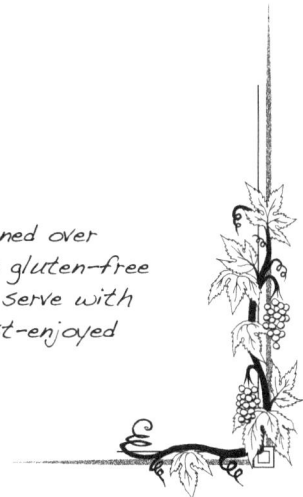

WHY GLUTEN-FREE?

Do you follow the gluten-free fad because you want to lose weight or have more energy? If so, you are on a dangerous path. Can you prove you are gluten-sensitive or intolerant? Have you consulted a gluten-sensitivity or celiac disease expert? If not, you are in danger of creating a bigger health issue for yourself than your present pain and discomfort. Dr. Osborne calls gluten sensitivity or intolerance a "state of genetics" and not a disease. Celiac is a disease. Sometimes, it takes from thirty to forty years for the symptoms of gluten sensitivity to surface.

It is essential to determine with as much accuracy as possible if you have an actual problem with gluten before you take on the gluten-free diet. Is something else going on? If you are certain you want to go for the diet, eliminate grains, beginning with wheat, a bit at a time. If you do it all at once, you can have a detox reaction, called the *Herxheimer Effect*, named after Jarisch-Herxheimer. It is a reaction to endotoxins released by the death of harmful organisms within the body. Another important step to remember is to read your labels carefully for toxic ingredients. Try the Elimination Diet.

"THE DIRTY LITTLE SECRET"

In a 2012 *New York Times Magazine*, Michael Pollen, popular chef and food expert, who has published books with cutting-edge information about nutrition and food, discussed the dangers of a gluten-free diet. He explains, "With all of the hype surrounding gluten-free, no one mentions the dirty little secret of the Standard Gluten-Free Diet. Few realize that when it comes to gluten-free baked goods such as bread, snacks, and desserts, gluten-free food is not as nutritious as 'regular' food."

Pollen continues with the idea that gluten-free goods are generally made with ingredients such as rice, corn, potatoes sorghum, tapioca and millet, which are higher in carbohydrates and lower in protein, and other ingredients, such as sugar, are less nutritious than wheat flour.

I agree with Pollen when he advises that the gluten-free diet is a very specific requirement for people with very specific symptoms of celiac disease, gluten intolerance, or gluten sensitivity. He also explains that it doesn't work to eliminate gluten without factoring in the entire range of healthy ingredients. He says we lose out if we think a gluten-free diet alone will cover the necessary nutritional elements we need in our diet and will cure all our other health problems.

My popular monthly lectures and consultations at Pharmaca Integrative Pharmacy in Pacific Palisades, California led to a collaboration that resulted in increased gluten-free store product sales. I taught their customers about gluten issues and was a keynote speaker for their annual Natural Children's Month. I repeat — I share my personal experience and my ongoing research. I don't diagnose or prescribe because everyone is different and our personal health solutions are always very individual. I encourage my clients and readers to listen to their body, their instinct, and intuition when they choose their food. Many Pharmaca customers had discovered these sensitivity issues by themselves, or had been diagnosed with related symptoms and wanted more information about the gluten-free fad. I love to share my experience and documented research whenever and wherever possible.

Even though the term *celiac* has become more familiar to many Americans, there is still a great deal of confusion about the truth about gluten sensitivity, intolerance, CD, and the gluten-free diet. Recently, the public's demand for more clarity and answers to the gluten dilemma has resulted in more in-depth research and documentation, which sometimes results in a vast amount of confusing information from the scientific and medical world. The answers to these questions vary from day to day. There is a rise in childhood diseases such as cancer and diabetes, and now, more mothers want to know which foods to feed their children so they will flourish. I have made a stab at answering some of the following questions in my book, because the grass-roots consumer has jumped onto the gluten-free bandwagon. Everyone who considers the gluten-free diet may want to clarify these questions for themselves:

- What is the truth about the gluten-free fad and gluten-free products?
- What does the term "Gluten-Free" really mean?
- Is a gluten-free regime just for celiacs?
- Is it harmful for people who are not gluten sensitive?
- Is it dangerous to go without grains?
- How long do I have to do this diet?

DANGEROUS OR SAFE?

Many people use the gluten-free fad as an excuse to lose weight without realizing the intricacies and threats to their health that are involved. Most of the processed and packaged "gluten-free" food products are toxic — many are GMO and contain corn, sugar, additives, are often cross-contaminated, and have cross-links. According to Dr. Osborne, we consume three thousand chemicals and additives a year if we eat packaged, processed foods, which means 150 pounds per person annually. Processed foods add GMO, herbicides, and pesticides to the mix, and our confused digestive systems begin to rebel and manufacture these same toxic bacteria as a defensive action. These dangerous toxins go directly to the liver, which is no longer able to detoxify, as it should.

Gluten issues may begin as a skin disorder such as acne or headaches and later manifest as cancer. Gluten affects each person in a different way, which sometimes makes gluten issues hard to detect and diagnose. It might be dangerous to go without grains if you don't have gluten issues. It depends on the individual. It sometimes takes thirty years of accumulated toxins to begin to manifest as a major disease. Many doctors now recommend going wheat-free, and don't have the necessary knowledge about gluten.

THE G-F FOOD PRODUCT CONFUSION

Most "gluten-free" products are usually made with high levels of carbohydrates and fructose. Carbohydrate overload is often the cause of diabetes and other metabolic disorders later in life.

When I discovered the gluten issue as Whole Foods Market's first food coach and consultant, I was new to the gluten issue. Although the gluten challenge was first researched fifty years ago, in 2010 there was a silent epidemic that had begun to engulf many people with wheat and gluten challenges. The gluten-free product boom began at a creep in 2005. By 2011 the gluten-free food industry, which began with small mom-and-pop businesses and individually owned health food stores, had become an international, multi-billion dollar business. Many major U.S. food corporations now run this mega-food business. In 2012, national supermarket chains jumped on the gluten-free podium as well, and some supermarkets now advertise G-F products and organic produce with their food discount coupons. In 2013 there was a five-billion dollar market for gluten-free processed foods.

GMO USA & OTHER COUNTRIES

In the past, the U.S. government subsidized farmers to grow corn and soy for worldwide export. Most of these farmers used GMO pesticides and other chemicals, which resulted in an agricultural disaster. The soil where these products grew was unsustainable, and diseases such as cancer and neurological diseases increased. In May, 2013, South Korea, and Japan refused U.S. tender for wheat because GMO, a chemical that the USDA termed illegal when it was developed in the 1950s, was found in their wheat shipments. As of 2013, China and the Philippines are still waiting for a valid test kit from the USDA. In 2014, Italy has the same issue in consideration awaiting the approval of three of their top governmental agencies. Many governments prefer to let their people go without because they don't want the GMO food products the USA offers them at a discount.

ARGENTINA

A Poster Child for the Health Hazards of GMO

- Massive spraying of herbicides on its genetically engineered Soya fields are sickening Argentina's population. Glyphosate, the main ingredient in Roundup™ (a Monsanto product), is blamed for the dramatic increase in devastating birth defects as well as cancer. Sterility and miscarriages are also increasing

- A 2012 nutritional analysis of GMO versus non-GMO corn shows shocking differences in nutritional content. Non-GMO corn contains 437 times more calcium, 56 times more magnesium, and 7 times more manganese than GMO corn

- GMO corn was also found to contain 13 ppm of glyphosate, compared to zero in non-GMO corn. The EPA standard for glyphosate in American water supplies is 0.7 ppm, and organ damage in animals has occurred at levels as low as 0.1 ppm

- GMO corn contains extremely high levels of formaldehyde—about 200 times the amount found toxic to animals

Dr Mercola Newsletter April 13, 2013

This USDA test kit is long overdue. Most of Western Europe has refused U.S. GMO grains for many years. Most of these GMO grains now go to Africa, because of their dire starvation issues; the result is protein deficiency there. A new study in the *American Journal of Preventive Medicine* concluded that U.S. agricultural policies contribute to America's general poor health, diabetes, and the obesity epidemic. The researchers wrote: "Government-issued payments have skewed agricultural markets toward the overproduction of commodities that are the basic ingredients of processed, energy-dense foods."

This includes corn, wheat, soybeans and rice, which are the top four most heavily subsidized foods. By subsidizing these products, particularly corn and soy, the U.S. government is actively supporting a diet that consists of these grains in their processed form, namely high-fructose corn syrup (HFCS), soybean oil, and grain-fed cattle — all of which are now well-known contributors to obesity and chronic diseases.

Dr. Mercola, in his free daily newsletter, writes that the USDA farm subsidy program subsidizes junk food in one federal office, while across the hall another department is funding an anti-obesity campaign. Farm subsidies bring you high-fructose corn syrup, fast food, junk food, CAFOs (concentrated animal feeding operations), monoculture, and a host of other contributors to our unhealthful contemporary diet.

He asks: why would a farmer choose to plant lettuce or Swiss chard when the government will essentially "insure" these GMO crops and pay them back if the market prices fall below a set floor price?

I repeat — when I teach or write I share my personal experience. I consider myself a researcher whose personal experience with some of the causes and answers for gluten issues is useful, not a nutritionist or therapist. Many people discover gluten-sensitivity issues by themselves, or have been diagnosed because of related symptoms. Once this autoimmune disease is diagnosed, it is easy to proceed toward symptom reduction and/or elimination. My main challenge is that many people, especially seniors, who have had the same basic diet for decades, are in denial about their eating habits. They don't want to change and don't know where and how to start the G-F regime.

I learned through my own experience with gluten sensitivity that we are all very unique when it comes to what we choose to eat and what we are willing to do to improve our health. I went cold turkey to avoid gluten because of my age and also because I had had cancer; I have immune system challenges due to chemo, radiation, and Tamoxifin. In general, however, it is safer to eliminate gluten one step at a time.

Gluten sensitivity is an autoimmune disease that causes inflammation, especially of the lower intestines. Gluten sensitivity also limits our ability to digest vitamin supplements. I took supplements for years and never noticed any major benefits until I eliminated gluten and started homeopathic, gluten-free supplements, Young Living essential oils, and the hair analysis.

We are what we eat and so many other issues influence our health. Our food choices and habits are reflected in our thoughts and feelings about our planet's environment, our societal and political issues, and our connection (or lack of connection) to Something Greater Than Ourselves, and our legacy.

When I went to Rome to help my ex-husband, Massimo through his final days of pancreatic cancer in May of 2010, I was surprised to see that the average Italian was very familiar with CD. Because Italians have some of the worst Celiac Disease on the planet, the Italian government requires school-age children to take a gluten intolerance test. Italian citizens are given a special discount on gluten-free products for their gluten-free diets. In 2013,

---

One of my favorite research sites, *About.com*,
published this survey in 2012:

Do you have an official diagnosis?

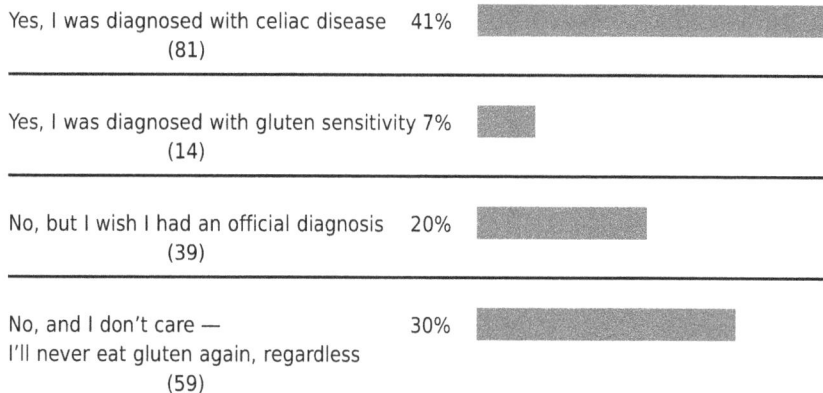

Yes, I was diagnosed with celiac disease (81)	41%	
Yes, I was diagnosed with gluten sensitivity (14)	7%	
No, but I wish I had an official diagnosis (39)	20%	
No, and I don't care — I'll never eat gluten again, regardless (59)	30%	

---

many North Americans are still in denial about wheat and gluten sensitivities. Due to the media attention (much of it false) on this topic, however, consumers have begun to accept the free brochures about this insidious disease that I'd tried to hand out (previously with little success) at farmers markets and businesses in the past. Beware of the gluten-free diet.

Doctors are hesitant to recommend this regime because they don't want to follow it themselves. Many in the medical and nutritional world see to avoid gluten and all grains are too complicated and "unappetizing." I learned through my own experience with gluten intolerance that we are all very unique when it comes to what we choose to eat and what we are willing to do to improve our health. After 10 years on a G-F regime, I learn something new on a daily basis, both because of my own body reactions to food intake and to the daily research I do about gluten.

RESEARCH

Melinda Beck observed in the *Wall Street Journal*, 3/15/11, that "Some experts think as many as 1 in 20 Americans may have some form of gluten sensitivity or intolerance, but there is no test or defined set of symptoms. The most common are IBS-like stomach problems, headaches, fatigue, numbness and depression." Peter Green, director of the Celiac Disease Center, says that "research into gluten sensitivity today is roughly where celiac disease was 30 years ago. Immune reactions were different, too. In the gluten-sensitive group, the response came from innate immunity, a primitive system with which the body sets up barriers to repel invaders. The subjects with celiac disease had less adaptive immunity, a more sophisticated system that develops specific cells to fight foreign bodies."

The findings still need to be replicated. It is still not understood how a reaction to gluten could cause such a wide range of symptoms. Many scientists believe a virus causes it. Dr. Fasano, a gluten challenge pioneer and expert, and others speculate that once immune cells are mistakenly primed to attack gluten, they can migrate and spread inflammation, even to the brain. Marios Hadjivassiliou, a neurologist in Sheffield, England, says he found deposits of antibodies to gluten in autopsies and brain scans of some patients with ataxia, a condition of impaired balance. Others have found it can be related to schizophrenia. Could such findings help explain why some parents of autistic,

ADHD, and ADD children say symptoms have improved—sometimes dramatically—when gluten was eliminated from their childrens' diets. To date, no scientific studies have emerged to back up such reports. Dr. Fasano hopes to eventually discover a biomarker specifically for gluten sensitivity. For now, a gluten-free diet is the only treatment recommended for gluten sensitivity, though some may be able to tolerate small amounts. I had the best results when I took all gluten away for two weeks and then put it back one ingredient at a time.

Tests are not as definitive for gluten as they are for wheat. Gluten affects different people in unpredictable ways and no tests are one hundred per-cent definitive at this time. Patients who receive a positive diagnosis are fortunate, because negative results often mean gluten is still lurking in the shadows and may surface at any time. Dr. Osborne's genetic test and a new patch test that is applied to the inside of the upper lip are hopeful.

For now, a gluten-free diet is the only treatment recommended for gluten sensitivity, though some may tolerate small amounts of gluten on occasion.

GET BACK TO NORMAL

How can you get back to "normal" after you've been glutened?

- Keep a strict G-F diet

- Take quick catnaps during the day. I often take three or four along with a few minutes of breathing exercises

- Do a tension-relieving exercise such as yoga

- Meditate

- Journal

- Use essential oils for relaxation. Apply them or diffuse them. I love Young Living Essential Oils, Release, Lavender, Digese and Frankincense

- Don't read newspapers or listen to the news before you sleep. You need as much deep sleep as possible.

> Mayo expert, Dr. Joseph Murray has researched the gluten issue for several years and lists several possible environmental causes of celiac disease:
>
> - *Over-clean environment (The immune system has little to attack and turns on itself)*
> - *Modern wheat hybridization and processing*
> - *The 21st century diet*
> - *The metabolic system processes wheat as sugar and over-consumption can begin an addiction similar to that of drugs and heroin.*

OTHER IDEAS

Something else to consider—the problem of toxic chemical exposure in American homes is reaching epidemic proportions. Americans are exposed to an average of 210,000 toxic chemicals every year that require medical treatment. These are exposures that can easily be eliminated with a little education and a resolve to make a difference.

I use the Young Living *Thieves Oil* Family Home Kit as the proven product to disinfect all home surfaces and to use when in public places to prevent flu and other infections (*www.youngliving.com*). I use their pure products for better digestion and to relieve stress and balance my emotions.

POSITIVITY AND DIGESTION

Barbara Fredrickson teaches in the psychology department of the University of Michigan. Her white paper, "The Broaden-and-Build Theory of Positive Emotions," published online August 17, 2004 offers valuable proof that positive emotions help us be more resilient and creative. My personal experience with emotions and eating proved to me that a positive attitude and mood always enhances my digestion, especially when I have a delicious meal at my favorite G-F restaurant and am confident I don't have to worry about gluten or allergy issues. When I am grumpy, I can be low on impulse control. If I don't monitor my mouth, I will grouch at the waitress or my dining companion.

I also learned in macrobiotics that your emotions affect the food you cook. The love and also the hate are passed on through the cook's energy.

Casey McCluskey's website *PositivelyPositive.com* is packed with excellent tips about health and vitality. She recommends these four steps to a better digestion for everyone:

1. Ensure you are sufficiently hydrated with pure water and fresh fruit and vegetable juices.

2. Eat when you're hungry and eat until satisfied, not stuffed.

3. Get your digestive enzymes.

4. Use herbs for digestive support.

I will add to this list the importance of a positive attitude and a commitment to your healthy eating habits.

BIG AGRICULTURE CAN DO NO WRONG

Monsanto Corp. Worthy of a "Nobel"... or the Booby Prize?

In 2012 President Obama signed into law a bill that included a devastating provision that puts biotech giant Monsanto above the law. The provision limits the ability of judges to stop Monsanto and/or farmers from growing or harvesting genetically engineered crops, even if courts find them to be toxic.

Ironically, Monsanto is under consideration at this time for half of a Nobel Prize award. On June 20, 2013 RT.com reported that the "Nobel of Agriculture" went to a Monsanto executive. Although not as high profile, the annual World Food Prize award, often referred to as the "Nobel Prize for Agriculture," and this year's winners — scientists with key roles in developing genetically engineered crops — may bring unwanted attention. The winners of the prize were announced at the U.S. State Department, with Secretary of State John Kerry in attendance. This year's award will be shared among three scientists: Marc Van Montague, Mary-Dell Chilton and Robert Fraley, all pioneers in agricultural biotechnology.

Fraley is currently the chief technology officer at Monsanto, while Mary-Dell Chilton is the founder of Syngenta Biotechnology, another prominent biotech company. In awarding the prize, which carries a $250,000 cash award, the Iowa-based World Food Prize Foundation temporized that genetically modified crops offer higher yields, and are more resilient to pestilence and adverse weather.[1]

As I review my gypsy travels through the various lands of diet and health regimes, I am pleased that I have taken responsibility for my daily diet in a way that works because I feel buoyant and healthy. I know, however, that my body always changes, especially as I age, and my health is something I want to monitor on a daily basis. I miss going out to eat, unless it is an authentic gluten-free restaurant, and I get tired of having to take my food with me when I go to a dinner party if the hostess doesn't know how to make one part of the dinner gluten-free.

I remember with nostalgia the sumptuous dinners I made in Italy and elsewhere, and all the exotic ingredients I used to eat. But I don't miss the arguments each mealtime when I tried to introduce certain products that enhanced the traditional Mediterranean Diet our family ate on a daily basis.

On the positive side, though, I am now healthier than I have ever been and have more energy and fewer mood swings. I get more accomplished as I conquer the gluten challenge each day.

I love to share my research and recipes with new and past acquaintances. To know that many mothers have become aware of the importance of nutrition and are more prepared to tailor delicious meals and to prevent toxic reactions to their family's diet gives me a glow. My childhood dream to change the world is coming true on a daily basis.

Food reflects our planet's ideals, values, ethics, morals, and desires. In this cookbook, I want my readers to take their daily eating patterns seriously. I also want to inspire my readers who are older, to share their new wisdom and knowledge as a gift to all those human beings they encounter who live on this magnificent planet. I want to help us all survive the increasing challenges we meet on a daily basis.

I encourage each reader to do their own research and use their common sense about their personal health issues. Have an open dialog with your doctors and nutrition experts and keep looking for answers that make sense when theirs don't satisfy you.

EAT REAL!

[1]*http://rt.com/usa/world-food-prize-monsanto-executive-971/*

10

ANCORA! COOK LIKE A PEASANT!

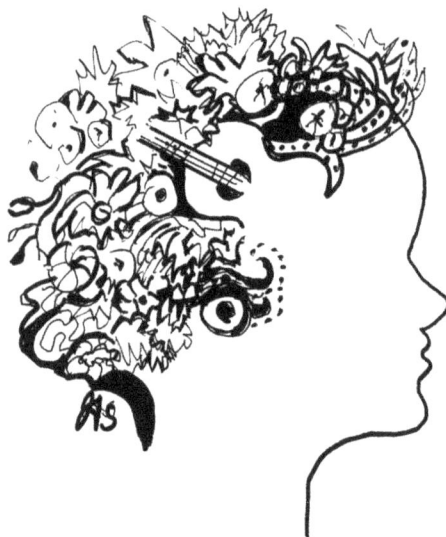

ILLUSTRATION BY JFS, AUTHOR

A TREASURY OF TRADITIONAL TUSCAN, GLUTEN-FREE RECIPES

As always, all vegetables should be organic and non-GMO or GE. Buy them from your local farmers market or grow them yourself whenever possible. Some of these recipes make fun gifts.

Olive and Caper Tapenade

Tapenades are perfect to keep on hand for unexpected guest treats, light meals, and snacks. Excellent on cheese and crackers, pasta, and for homemade gifts any time of the year. Add some to Chevre or serve it alongside Manchego or Gouda goat cheese. It also makes superb grilled cheese sandwiches with Monterey Jack or Gruyere cheese.

INGREDIENTS

½ lb. (1½ cups) pitted, organic black or green olives (such as Kalamata or green Sicilian), rinsed and drained

2 Tbsp. capers, rinsed and drained

3 anchovy fillets, rinsed and patted dry

2 medium cloves garlic, smashed and peeled

1 teaspoon Dijon mustard

1½ Tbsp. fresh lemon juice

1 Tbsp. extra-virgin olive oil

1 Tbsp. finely chopped fresh flat-leaf parsley

PREPARATION

Put the olives, capers, anchovies, garlic, and mustard in a food processor and pulse until smooth. With the motor running, add the lemon juice and oil. Transfer to a bowl and stir in the parsley and ¼ teaspoon of pepper.

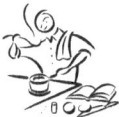

Tapenade can be refrigerated in an airtight container for up to one month.

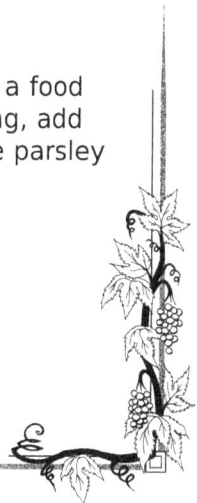

Chef's Note

CHRISTINA'S SPICED GARBANZOS (CHICKPEAS)

*I adapted this recipe to be gluten-free from my friend who lives in Topanga
Canyon, California. She is a very creative entrepreneur who loves good
food and likes to cook. Christina and her husband travel the world for
their business and enjoy this recipe and a good glass of wine when
they entertain at their beautiful home.*

INGREDIENTS

2 15oz cans of organic chickpeas
2 Tbsp. organic olive oil
1½ Tbsp. organic coconut sugar
1 teaspoon smoked paprika
1 teaspoon Cajun seasoning
½ teaspoon Himalayan salt
¼ teaspoon cayenne pepper
¼ teaspoon red pepper flakes

PREPARATION

Preheat oven to 425° F.

Mix all ingredients together and put on a roasting pan and roast
until crunchy.

Drain on a paper towel and serve hot or at room temperature

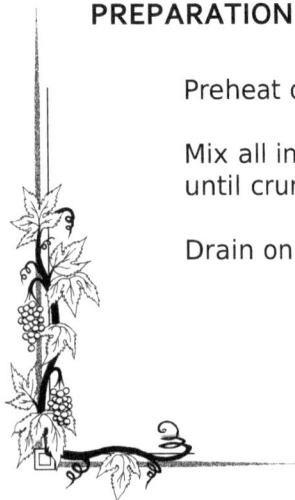

Honeyed Cipollini (TINY ONIONS)

These tiny onions are fun to keep on hand. You can add them to martinis or eat them as an accompaniment to any roast. I put them on fancy toothpicks and stick them in a half grapefruit or an apple. You can find the peeled onions in vinegar at a specialty store or online and add the other ingredients.

Cipollini are best the next day served with grilled or poached meat, fowl, or fish. They are perfect for gypsy picnics and keep well in your caravan's refrigerator.

For more simple onions, just cook in white wine, olive oil, salt and a bay leaf. Stir in honey at the end when the liquid is cool.

INGREDIENTS

½ lb. peeled, small, organic boiling onions
1 red chili pepper flakes (optional)
1 Tbsp. olive oil
1 Tbsp. tomato paste

Water and/or white wine
Himalayan salt
2 Tbsp. apple cider vinegar
2 Tbsp. raw honey

PREPARATION

Place onions in a single layer in a large, flat sauté pan. Cover with the white wine, diluted with water.

Add red chili pepper flakes, vinegar, olive oil, salt, and tomato paste. Stir to mix.

Cover and simmer for 10 minutes stirring occasionally until the water is gone.

Stir occasionally to prevent burning or sticking.

Cool and add raw honey. Mix well and remove red chili before serving. Taste to balance the sweet and sour flavors.

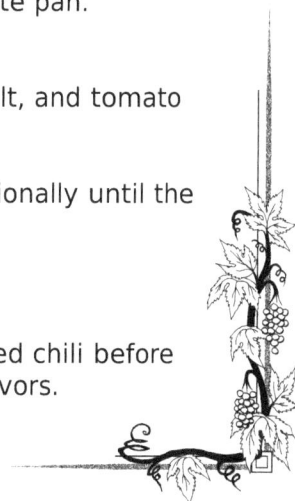

URBAN GYPSY WILD MUSHROOM SOUP

*Urban Gypsies forage for organic 'shrooms in farmers markets, online,
in the forest, and other wild locations. Dried, wild mushrooms also work
for this recipe. Soak in warm water or wine, strain, and lift the soaking
liquid off to add to the broth, being careful not to disturb the residue.*

INGREDIENTS

1½ Tbsp. grape seed oil

1 large shallot, minced

3 cups dried wild mushrooms, soaked, softened, and strained

1 large, organic Portobello mushroom, chopped

1 teaspoon organic, fresh rosemary, minced

1 teaspoon organic fresh sage, minced

Black pepper

⅓ cup dry Marsala or red wine

2 cups organic low-salt chicken broth

1 Tbsp. olive oil

1 oz. finely grated Parmigiano-Reggiano (1 cup using a rasp grater)
(optional)

¼ cup crème fraîche or heavy cream

¼ cup Italian parsley chopped

Himalayan salt

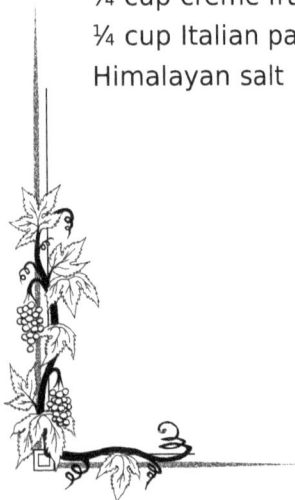

PREPARATION

Heat the grapeseed oil in a 4-quart saucepan over medium heat.

Add the shallot, ½ teaspoon salt and sauté, stirring, until shallot begins to brown at the edges, 3 to 4 minutes.

Add the wild and Portobello mushrooms and herbs, 1½ teaspoon salt, and ¼ teaspoon pepper.

Increase the heat to medium high, and cook, stirring, until the mushrooms soften and start to brown, 3 to 5 minutes.

Add the Marsala and stir until reduced by half, about 2 minutes.

Add the broth and 1 cup water; bring to a boil. Reduce the heat and simmer for 5 minutes.

Working in batches, purée the soup in a blender until smooth.

Transfer to a 3-quart saucepan and reheat.

Add olive oil and parsley.

In a small bowl, mix the crème fraîche and chives.

Season the soup to taste with salt and serve topped with a swirl of the crème fraîche and a sprinkling of Parmesan

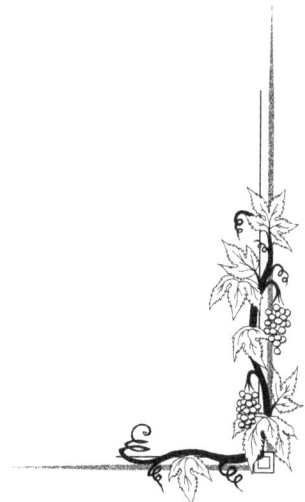

PERPETUAL BONE BROTH — THE EASY WAY

This is another "in bianco" (white dish), and a popular recipe all over Europe because it is very nutritious, good for invalids, and economical. You can make enough of this mineral-rich broth to last for a week. At the end a week's simmering, strain off any remaining broth and discard or compost the bones. Cool the broth and refrigerate. Skim off the fat that rises to the top and use it for cooking other dishes. Freeze the broth for the future.

INGREDIENTS

1 whole, organic chicken or the frame of a roasted chicken
2 sweet bay leaves
Whole, organic root vegetables or scraps
Filtered water

GLUTEN-FREE KETCHUP

This also makes a good G-F BBQ sauce with the addition of Worstershire sauce, Dijon mustard, and organic coconut sugar.

INGREDIENTS

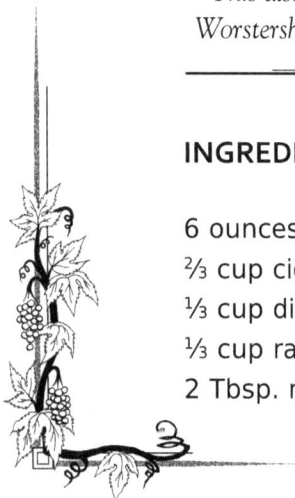

6 ounces tomato paste
⅔ cup cider vinegar
⅓ cup distilled water
⅓ cup raw honey
2 Tbsp. minced onions

2 cloves garlic
1 teaspoon Himalayan salt
⅛ teaspoon ground allspice
⅛ teaspoon ground cloves
⅛ teaspoon black pepper

PREPARATION

Place one whole chicken or the frame of a roasted chicken into your slow cooker with sweet bay, black peppercorns and any vegetable scraps you have on hand. Cover with filtered water and cook on low for one week.

After twenty-four hours, you may begin using the broth.

As you need broth or stock, simply dip a ladle or measuring cup into the slow cooker to remove the amount of stock you need.

Pour it through a fine-mesh sieve or, preferably, a reusable coffee filter, which will help to clarify the broth. Replace the broth you remove from the slow cooker with an equivalent amount of filtered water.

At the end of the week, strain off any remaining broth and discard or compost the bones. The bones from your chicken should crumble when pressed between your thumb and forefinger. Their softness is an indication that much of the nourishment from the bones — minerals, amino acids — have leached from the bones and into the broth you've enjoyed all week long. Wash the insert of your slow cooker and start again.

PREPARATION

Put everything in your blender and run it until the onion disappears.

Scrape into a container with a tight lid and store in the refrigerator.

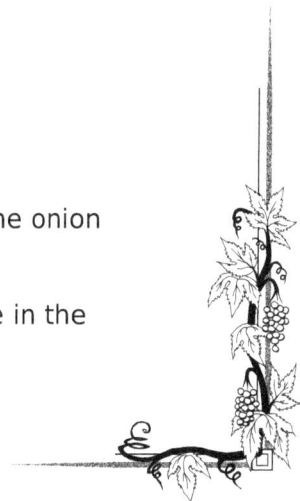

ZIO (UNCLE) TEBALDO'S SECRET HERB MIX

These herbs and spices were the secret recipe of Zio Tebaldo, who lived in Cireglio, a tiny village in the mountains of the Tuscan Dolomites. Zio Tebaldo was short, wiry, very strong, and very secretive. He and his family had lived there for centuries, and his wife, Zia Lorena, was one of the best home cooks I ever met. Tebaldo taught me how to hunt for Porcini mushrooms… the best-tasting mushrooms that Tuscans value more than their famous Bistecca Fiorentina (T-Bone steak), We would go out with a flashlight while it was still dark. Tebaldo carried a rifle, as he didn't want anyone poaching his secret mushroom treasure trove. We would bring the mushrooms back in an ancient basket, full to the brim. Lorena would make polenta and roast a rabbit Tebaldo had shot… a dinner fit for royalty. Tuscans say, "Cook like a peasant and dine like royalty."

Our menu was polenta with Porcini mushroom sauce, roast rabbit, and homegrown wild arugula salad. Lorena would always have a pie waiting baked with fruit from their trees: peaches, plums, apples, or pears. Dinner would end with a typical Tuscan Biscotti di Prato, espresso, and Sambuca liqueur.

INGREDIENTS

¼ cup dried sage
¼ cup dried rosemary
1 bay leaf
⅛ cup grated lemon peel

1 Tbsp. juniper berries
2 Tbsp. garlic powder
1 Tbsp. black pepper
1 teaspoon quality salt

PREPARATION

Mix all the ingredients well and put in a jar. Use a tablespoon at a time for roasts, stews, soups, and anything else your imagination can come up with. I sometimes put it in a soft goat cheese and eat it with organic Granny Smith apples or pears.

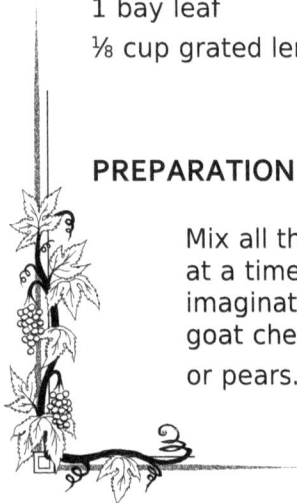

Pollo al Principe: a Florentine Prince's Chicken Breast

SERVES 4

*I adapted this recipe to gluten-free from my longtime friend from Rome,
Loretta Holliday, who tasted it at a Florentine Prince's invitation many years ago.
We raised our infant sons together in Rome, and we Skype from Topanga to North
Carolina now. We still love to exchange recipes and reminisce about our days in Italy
and both of our sons, Sacha and Patrick, who are successful young men in their late 40s.*

INGREDIENTS

1 Tbsp. organic grapeseed oil

1 Tbsp. organic, cultured, unsalted butter

3 cloves organic garlic, minced

½ cup coconut or almond flour

Himalayan salt

1 Tbsp. sage and/or rosemary, minced, or ½ Tbsp. dried leaves,
   or ground Red pepper flakes

4 organic, boneless chicken breasts

1 cup organic white wine, or Marsala,

Juice of one organic, fresh squeezed lemon

3 cloves organic garlic, minced

½ cup Italian parsley, chopped

PREPARATION

Sprinkle breasts with salt and red pepper flakes.
Blend flour and herbs.
Coat breasts with flour and shake off remaining flour.
Sauté in a large, heavy skillet in grapeseed oil and butter
until golden on both sides and almost done.
Sprinkle with finely minced garlic.
Add wine or lemon juice and reduce to a glaze.
Garnish with giant caper berries and Italian parsley.

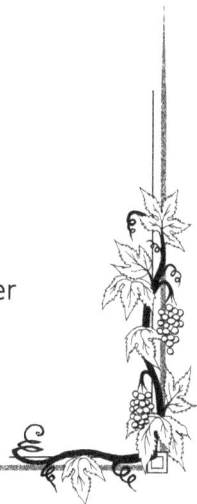

HUNTER'S ROAST RABBIT

SERVES 4

Urban gypsies hunt their rabbits at the butcher's instead of the forest.
Europeans love game and savor the taste and protein of a good hare or
rabbit. Americans are pften more squeamish about eating a bunny because
they keep them as pets, however, rabbit meat is becoming more popular
of late. Be sure your rabbit and ingredients are all organic!

This is a classic Tuscan recipe for roasts. Use it with a beef or lamb roast
or root vegetables and. Use with Uncle Tebaldo's Secret Herb Mix (page 154)
It is also delicious cold and perfect for a light "in bianco" meal or a picnic.

INGREDIENTS

2½ to 2¾ pound rabbit in one piece

2 large cloves garlic, split

1 stick unsalted butter, at room temperature, or 6 tablespoons
   extra-virgin olive oil

Himalayan salt and lemon pepper

1 inch sprig fresh rosemary, or ½ teaspoon dried rosemary leaves

6 fresh sage leaves or 1 teaspoon dried sage

6 juniper berries

½ cup dry white wine

3 Tbsp. fresh lemon juice

3 to 4 sprigs fresh rosemary for garnish

PREPARATION

Roasting the Rabbit: Preheat oven to 325 degrees.

Rinse and dry the rabbit thoroughly. Rub it all over with the
split garlic and reserve the garlic. Slather the entire surface
of the rabbit with the butter or olive oil.

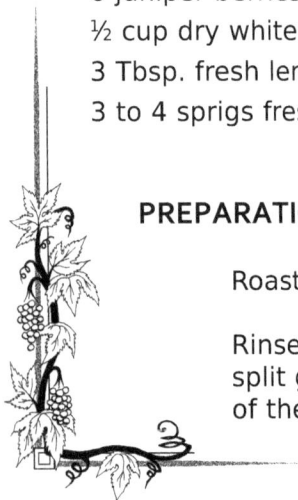

Place the rabbit in a large, shallow roasting pan.

Sprinkle on all sides with salt and pepper. Add the garlic and herbs to the pan.

Roast for 30 minutes before pouring the wine and lemon juice over it.

Spoon the pan juices over the meat, cover loosely with foil, and continue roasting l hour.

Every 15 minutes give the rabbit a quarter turn and baste with the pan juices. Then turn heat up to 450 degrees and uncover rabbit.

Roast another 15 minutes, or until deep golden brown. Baste often with the pan juices to keep meat succulent, and turn once or twice for even coloring.

Have a warm serving platter ready. Use poultry shears to cut rabbit into serving pieces.

Arrange on the platter with sprigs of rosemary and sage. Drizzle the rabbit with its pan juices, if desired.

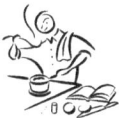

Chef's Note

Roast and eat immediately. It will hold, lightly covered with foil, in a turned-off oven about 15 minutes

Serve the rabbit with garlicky mashed potatoes and roast fennel. You can roast the fennel in the pan with the rabbit.

Special order your rabbit from your butcher or market

This is a classic Tuscan recipe for roasts. Use it with a beef or lamb roast or vegetables.

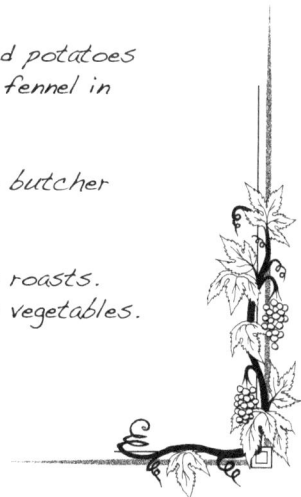

Veal Marsala

SERVES 4

This recipe is a surefire way to please your dinner guests that also is delicious with chicken breast fillets. Have your butcher slice the veal very thin and don't overcook it or it will be dry. Serve it with an Orvieto or any other dry, white wine, and artichokes with a lemon-butter sauce.

INGREDIENTS

3 Tbsp. organic unsalted butter, divided

1 Tbsp. grapeseed oil

1 pound Portobello mushrooms, quartered

2 large garlic clove, minced

1½ pound veal cutlets (also called scaloppini; ¼-inch thick)

½ teaspoon Himalayan salt

¼ teaspoon black pepper

½ teaspoon dried organic rosemary, minced and divided

½ teaspoon dried organic sage, minced and divided

⅓ cup almond flour

1 Tbsp. grapeseed oil

1½ Tbsp. olive oil

⅔ cup dry Marsala wine

1 cup beef or veal demiglace*

½ cup Italian parsley

PREPARATION

Heat 2 tablespoons butter in a 12-inch heavy skillet over high heat until foam subsides, then sauté mushrooms, stirring frequently, until liquid mushrooms give off is evaporated and mushrooms begin to brown, about 10 minutes.

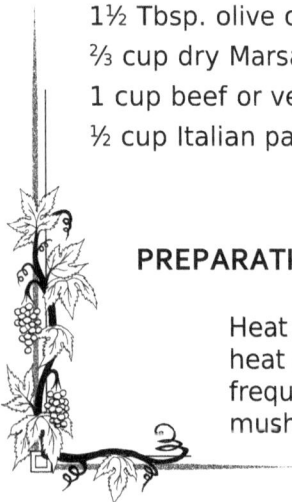

Add garlic and herbs, and sauté, stirring, 1 minute. Transfer to a bowl and wipe skillet clean. Remove to a bowl and keep warm.

Pat veal dry, and then sprinkle with salt, pepper and herbs.

Heat ½ tablespoon grapeseed oil with 1 teaspoon butter in skillet over moderately high heat until hot but not smoking.

While fat is heating, quickly dredge 2 or 3 pieces of veal in flour, shaking off excess, then sauté until just cooked through, 1 to 1 ½ minutes on each side (meat will still be slightly pink inside).

Transfer to a platter with tongs and keep warm, loosely covered. Sauté remaining veal in 2 more batches using remaining oil and butter.

Add Marsala to skillet and deglaze by boiling, stirring and scraping up brown bits, until reduced by half. Stir in demiglace and simmer, stirring occasionally, 2 minutes.

Stir in mushroom mixture and any veal juices accumulated on platter, then season with salt and pepper if necessary.

Simmer 2 minutes more, Sprinkle with Italian parsley and spoon over veal.

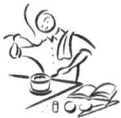

Chef's Note

We use Demi-Glace Gold, available in specialty foods shops, and some supermarkets

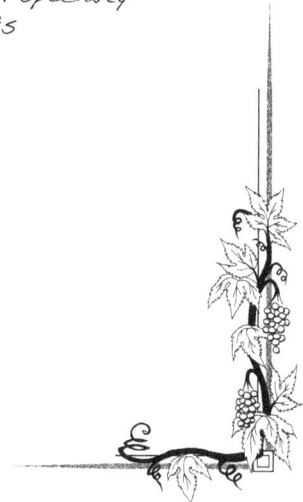

Mamma Bianca's Chicken Piccatta

SERVES 4

Forty years ago, I tasted this recipe in Modena (home of Balsamic Vinegar). It was at lunch at an ancient Countess's table and was served with asparagus from her garden, Prosecco, and strawberries in red wine. Everything was cooked in butter. My mother-in-law, Bianca, served it as a light meal for hot summer days. Both dishes still make my mouth water. They are delicious cold or at room temperature and perfect for picnics.

Have your butcher slice the chicken breast into thin scaloppini and be sure to shake off all the flour before you sauté them. I like to brine my chicken in salt for a few hours before I cook them. Be sure to pat them dry and use less salt when you cook them.

INGREDIENTS :

4 organic, boneless chicken breasts
4 teaspoon almond flour
Himalayan salt and pepper
2 Tbsp. grapeseed oil, divided
1 medium shallot, minced
1 clove garlic
2 Tbsp. capers, drained and rinsed
½ cup organic, GF chicken broth
¼ cup lemon juice
½ cup fresh, organic Italian parsley, chopped

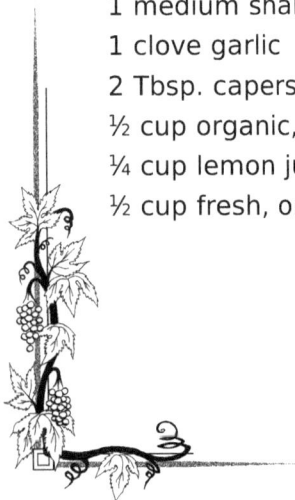

PREPARATION

Mix tapioca starch and almond flour into a shallow dish.
Season chicken with salt and pepper then dredge in flour mixture.

Heat 1 Tbsp. oil in cast iron skillet and fry chicken until golden,
fully cooked, and crispy. Set aside and tent to keep warm.

Heat 1 Tbsp. grapeseed oil in skillet and sauté shallot until soft.
Be careful not to burn.

Stir in capers, broth, and lemon juice. Stir, scraping any browned
bits into sauce.

If want a thicker sauce, add a tapioca mixture (2 teaspoons
tapioca starch and 2 teaspoons cold water) into the skillet,
stirring well.

Remove from heat and stir in parsley.

Pour sauce over chicken and sprinkle with parsley.

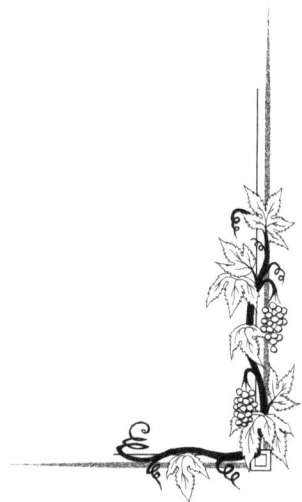

FIGS IN MARSALA SAUCE

SERVES 4

Massimo and I had impromptu dinners a few times a week when my husband would bring home out of work actors or directors at the last minute. This is a dessert you can make a week ahead and have on hand. My cooking school students and catering clients love it! This recipe also works well with ripe peaches and pears. Add raisins for extra sweetness or a raspberry coulis sauce. You can serve it either cold, room temperature, or warm. It's the perfect dessert for any season.

INGREDIENTS :

2 cups sweet Marsala wine
24 dried figs or fresh figs with stems on
2 Tbsp. fresh rosemary leaves, minced
1 cup raw honey

PREPARATION

Bring Marsala to a boil and then lower heat to a simmer.

Add figs and rosemary.

Turn the heat as low as possible and cover. Simmer gently until soft.

Stir occasionally to make sure the figs are submerged in the sauce; don't overcook the fresh figs.

Remove figs with a slotted spoon and turn the heat to medium-high; reduce the liquid to about half.

Mix the raw honey with the Marsala.

Pour the syrup over the prunes and chill or serve warm with marscarpone, whipped cream, or gluten-free ice cream and biscotti.

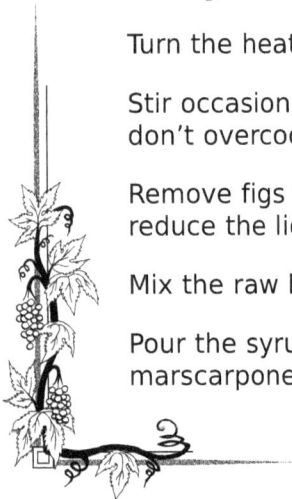

ROAST DUCK WITH POMEGRANATE REDUCTION

SERVES 2

I never had duck in Italy; however, melegrani (pomegranates) are plentiful in the autumn and winter season, and are served this way in restaurants that specialize in game.

My mother hated to cook anything; yet, a simple roast duck or two was always on her menu to cook for our family dinner parties. She served it every year for Thanksgiving and the Christmas season, (even though we were Jewish,) and her reputation benefited as Sarabelle's Roast Duck became a family tradition. We had sparkling Portuguese rose, my Grandma Fanny's Waldorf salad, canned cranberry sauce, and Grandma Fanny's pineapple and whipped cream fool with crispy butter cookies for a light dessert. My mouth waters just to remember it.

I roast duck breast or legs as a treat for myself. I find them at the market in packages and use this same recipe. So special and tasty! I prefer duck rare and like it cold for warm weather lunches and outings. Try Uncle Tebaldo's Secret Herbs in this chapter for a different roast rub.

INGREDIENTS

1 organic duck (4–5 pounds)
4 cloves organic garlic
1 Tbsp. organic fresh rosemary, mined
1 Tbsp. organic fresh sage, mined
1 Tbsp. juniper berries, crushed
1 organic orange, halved
1 yellow onion coarsely chopped
2 stalks celery cut into quarter strips
2 bay leaves
2 teaspoons quality salt
1 teaspoon pepper

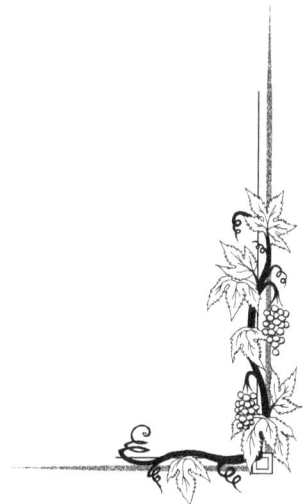

PREPARATION

<u>First Method</u>

Pre-heat oven to 475° F.

Cut the duck in half. Remove backbone, neck, and wing tips.

Place onions, celery, and bay leaves in a small roasting pan.

Place duck halves, cut side down on the bed of vegetables.

Prick duck skin all over with a fork. Rub with sea salt and pepper.

Insert orange halves in duck cavity.

Roast for 15 minutes at 475°, remove from the oven, prick skin again, cover with aluminum foil, reduce heat to 275, and roast for 3–4 hours.

Remove duck from the oven, reserve 2 tablespoons of duck fat, and turn on the broiler.

Cut the duck into quarters, place on a shallow baking sheet, and broil 10 inches from the heating element for 5 minutes.

(You can roast the duck earlier in the day and broil just before serving, but bring the duck to room temperature first)

<u>Second Method</u>

This method is more complicated, but still easy to make. The duck is cooked in half the time, so will be medium rare with a crusty skin. It takes longer to marinate, but the result is a more sophisticated dish.

This works well for duck breasts and legs. Just rub the spice over the meat and air dry for 24 hours.

Mix garlic, herbs, salt, pepper, and berries.

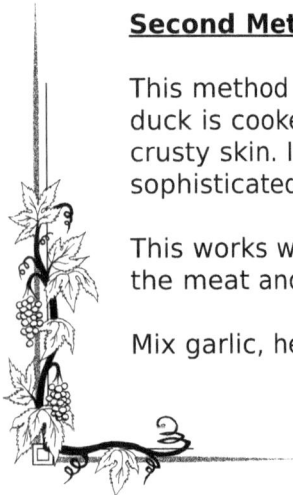

Make 20 to 30 small slits in the skin of the duck, using a sharp paring knife held parallel to the duck surface so that you pierce the skin and fat but not the meat. Be sure to make slits on the backs and thighs as well as the breasts when you use a whole duck.

Rub about two-thirds of the spice mixture into the duck cavity and then rub the remaining all over the skin. Insert the orange halves into the duck cavity. Set the ducks on a rack over a large rimmed baking sheet and allow to air dry uncovered in the refrigerator for 24 to 36 hours.

Roast the Duck

Position a rack in the center of the oven and heat the oven to 325°F.

Let the ducks sit at room temperature as the oven heats.

Arrange the ducks breast down on two small V-racks in a large roasting pan and roast for 1¼ hours.

Remove the pan from the oven and spoon or pour off most of the fat from the roasting pan — use a turkey baster if you have one. Flip the duck, using sturdy tongs inserted in the cavities, and pierce the skin again all over with a knife.

Continue roasting the duck until the meat around the thighs feels tender when prodded (a skewer should penetrate the thigh with no resistance), the legs feel loose in their joints, and an instant-read thermometer inserted in the thickest part of the thigh near the joint reads 175°F, 45 to 60 minutes more.

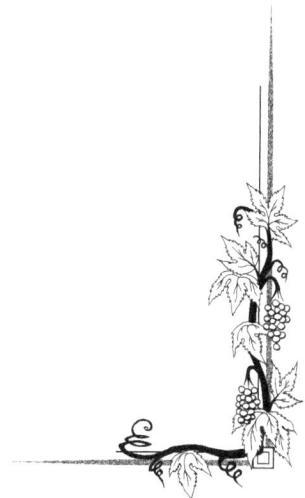

POMEGRANATE REDUCTION

INGREDIENTS

2 cups pomegranate juice

2 cups chicken broth (or you can make your own duck broth from wing tips and neck)

2 teaspoons white wine vinegar

2 Tbsp. organic coconut sugar

16–20 black peppercorns

2 packed teaspoons lemon zest

2 medium shallots sliced

2 teaspoons olive oil

2 Tbsp. almond flour

½ cup pomegranate seeds for garnish

PREPARATION

Sauté and caramelize shallots in olive oil (15 minutes).

Add juice, broth, vinegar, sugar, peppercorns, and zest.

Bring to boil, and then reduce heat to low. Maintain slow rolling boil on low heat for 50 minutes until the sauce is reduced to about a cup of liquid. Strain the sauce.

Make roux with 2 tablespoons each of flour and duck fat and whisk in sauce over medium heat until it starts to thicken.

Place duck in serving platter, pour sauce over it, and garnish with pomegranate seeds.

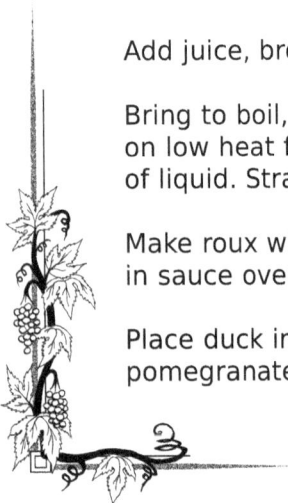

Fiori Fritti: Fried Zucchini Blossoms

These summertime flowers could also be called "Fairy Flowers" because they are so delicate and full of magic. They can be eaten as an antipasto, side dish, or sautéed and added to a frittata for a picnic. Fry them in coconut or grapeseed oil as olive oil is not good for frying and would be too heavy. Have your dinner guests at a casual party fry their own and eat them right away as an appetizer. This is a treat for the Gods!

Female zucchini produce flowers and males do not. The blossoms are wide open in the early morning sun and that is when you should pick them. The blossoms can be simply fried as a side dish or to make them richer, fill with ricotta cheese or day-old mozzarella cubes and pieces of anchovy.

INGREDIENTS FOR BATTER

1 cup of almond flour
¼ cup coconut flour
1 egg white
½ cup milk, coconut milk, or white wine
Pinch of sea salt
Pinch nutmeg, grated
Grapeseed or coconut oil for frying

PREPARATION

Stir above ingredients except egg white, until smooth and not too thick. *If it is too thick, thin with a little more milk or wine.*

Whisk the egg white until light and fluffy as for a meringue Stir in small amount to lighten the mixture then fold in the rest.

Heat oil for frying.

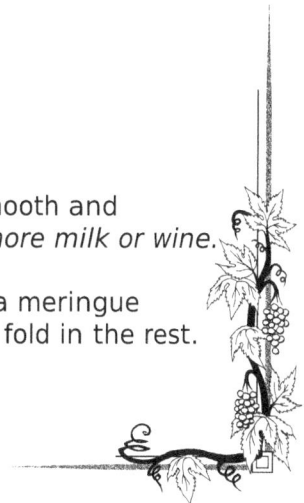

Dip the blossoms in the batter to cover completely and fry immediately.

I turn a couple of times with a fork to make sure they are crispy.

Lay on paper towel to drain and lightly salt or sugar before serving.

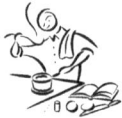

Chef's Note

Best eaten right out of the pan.

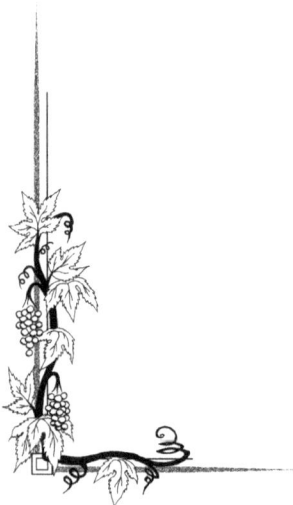

11

RESOURCES

THE CARAVAN MOVES ONWARD

CELIAC ORGANIZATIONS

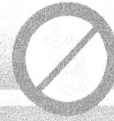

American Celiac Society – (ACS)   Phone: 973-325-8837

59 Crystal Avenue
West Orange, NJ 07052

E-mail: info@americanceliacsociety.org
Internet: http://williamshaffer.org/acs/

American Dietetic Association – (ADA)   Phone: 1-800-366-1655
or 1-800-877-1600

120 South Riverside Plaza, Suite 2000
Chicago, IL 60606-6995

E-mail: hotline@eatright.org
Internet: http://www.eatright.org

Celiac.com   Phone: 707-509-4528
Fax: 707-324-6060

P.O. Box 279
Gardena, CA 90248

E-mail: orders@celiac.com
Internet: http://www.celiac.com

Celiac Disease Foundation – (CDF)   Phone: 818-990-2354
Fax: 818-990-2379

13251 Ventura Boulevard, Suite #1
Studio City, CA 91604-1838

E-mail: cdf@celiac.org
Internet: http://www.celiac.org

Celiac Sprue Association – USA, Inc. – (CSA–USA)   Phone: 1-877-272-4272
or 402-558-0600
Fax: 402-558-1347

P.O. Box 31700
Omaha, NE 68131-0700

E-mail: celiacs@csaceliacs.org
Internet: http://www.csaceliacs.org

Gluten Intolerance Group of North America – (GIG)   Phone: 206-246-6652
Fax: 206-246-6531

15110 10th Avenue, SW., Suite A
Seattle, WA 98166

E-mail: info@gluten.net
Internet: http://www.gluten.net

Gluten-Free Living – (GFL)   Phone: 914-969-2018
(a bimonthly newsletter)

P.O. Box 105
Hastings-on-Hudson, NY 10706

E-mail: gfliving@aol.com
Internat: http://www.glutenfreeliving.com/

National Foundation for Celiac Awareness – (NFCA)   Phone: 215-325-1306
124 South Maple Street
Ambler, PA 19002

E-mail: info@celiacawareness.org
Internat:http://www.celiacawareness.org

**North American Society for Pediatric Gastroenterology,
Hepatology and Nutrition — (NASPGHAN)**   Phone: 215-233-0808

P.O. Box 6
Flourtown, PA 19031

E-mail: naspghan@naspghan.org
Internet: http://www.naspghan.org, or http://www.cdhnf.org

National Digestive Disease Information Clearinghouse – (NDDIC)
2 Information Way
Bethesda, MD 20892-3570

E-mail: nddic@info.niddk.nih.gov

WebMD - MedicineNet.com
(Celiac Disease)

Internet: http://www.medicinenet.com/celiac_disease/article.htm

---

The Israeli Celiac Association   Phone: 972-3-678-1481
Internet: http://www.celiac.org.il/

(in Hebrew – some English information)

FOOD PROTECTIVE AGENCIES

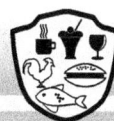

Below are some U.S. food agencies to contact for research and questions:

FDA Meat and Poultry Hotline   800-332-4010

FDA Seafood Hotline   800-332-4010

USDA Meat and Poultry Hotline   888-674-6854
                                                 mphotline.fsis@usda.gov

USDA Information Hotline   202-720-2791

Food Democracy Now   917-968-7369
                                                 dave@fooddemocracynow.org

FSIS   202-720-9113
                                                 NACMPI@fsis.usda.gov
                                                 mphotline.fsis@usda.gov

The Cornucopia Institute   608-625-2000
   Farmers, consumers, stakeholders involved in the good food movent, and the media
                                                 www.cornucopia.com

Sustainable Harvest
                                                 http://www.sustainableharvest.org

The Sustainable Food Trade Association
                                                 http://www.sustainablefoodtrade.org/

FOOD HEALTH ADVICE WEBSITES

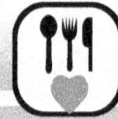

www.rodalenews.com	**celiacdisease.about.com**
www.rodalenews.com	**www.farmtoconsumer.org/**
www.savoryinstitute.com	**www.nourishingourchildren.org**
www.oxfamamerica.org	**www.nokidhungry.org**
feedingamerica.org/foodbank	**ppnf.org**

Dr. Peter Osborne   281-240-2229
Free Newsletter: *glutenology@gmail.com*

E-mail: support@glutenfreesociety.org

Gluten-Free Gift Labels

Labels that are great for your jars and bottles. I store and freeze everything in glass containers and love to give food gifts with some extra labels as gifts. I put them on my homemade food gifts to support and educate my friends and family about gluten-free foods and how delicious they can be.

www.Gluten-freelabels.com

GlutenFree (an Israeli Gluten-Free Market)

972-3-9191025
Fax: 972-3-9191026
P.O.B 65 Kokhav Yair 44864, Israel
Ware House: 6 Ha'mefalsim St. Kiryat Aria
Petach Tikva
Israel
Hours: (Sun-Thu 10:00-20:00, Fri 09:00-13:00)
E-mail:info@glutenfree.co.il
Internet: http://www.glutenfree.co.il/
(in Hebrew — click Amer. flag icon for English page)

Gluten-Free Living – (GFL)   914-969-2018
(a bimonthly newsletter)

P.O. Box 105
Hastings-on-Hudson, NY 10706

E-mail: gfliving@aol.com
http://www.glutenfreeliving.com/Internat:

SUSTAINABLE FOOD RESOURCES

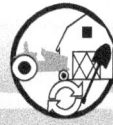

www.localharvest.org

Local Harvest — This Web site will help you find farmers' markets, family farms, and other sources of sustainably grown food in your area where you can buy produce, grass-fed meats, and many other goodies.

www.ams.usda.gov/farmersmarkets

Farmers' Markets — A national listing of farmers' markets.

www.eatwellguide.org

Eat Well Guide: Wholesome Food from Healthy Animals — The Eat Well Guide is a free online directory of sustainably raised meat, poultry, dairy, and eggs from farms, stores, restaurants, inns, and hotels, and online outlets in the United States and Canada.

www.buylocalfood.org

Community Involved in Sustaining Agriculture (CISA) — CISA is dedicated to sustaining agriculture and promoting the products of small farms.

www.foodroutes.org

FoodRoutes — The FoodRoutes "Find Good Food" map can help you connect with local farmers to find the freshest, tastiest food possible. On their interactive map, you can find a listing for local farmers, CSAs, and markets near you.

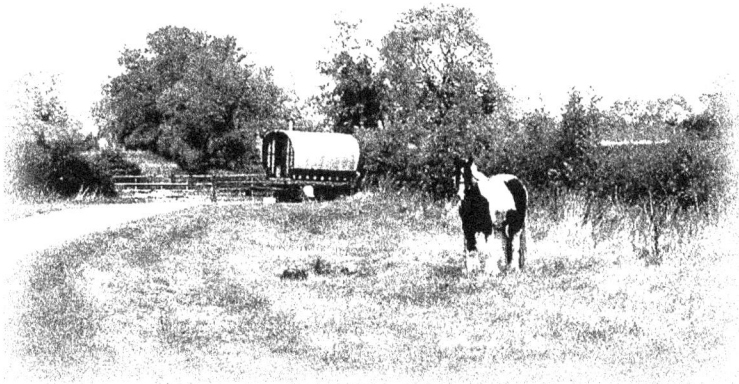

READER'S NOTES

CONTACT THE AUTHOR

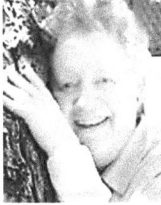

For more information about The Family Meal Program or marketing coaching, send an email to *sarchjudith@gmail.com* or *info@judithsarchielli.com* and let me know if the information presented in this book has been helpful. Please tell me about your personal experiences with a gluten-free diet or celiac disease.

Sound Nutrition Is the First Step on a Path to Health ...But Every Path Still Needs a Destination.

Do You Have a Clearly Visualized Goal for Your Life?

Along with providing sound nutritional advice and creating and teaching recipes based on the centuries-old Tuscan Cuisine, I have also been helping people design their lives and their businesses through the use of VISUALIZATION SOLUTIONS, using Vision Boards to map your life's possibilities.

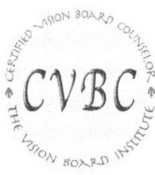

As a Certified Vision Board Counselor, I want to guide you to focus your intentions and realize your goals through the use of visualization techniques that will help to open new doors, find new pathways and tune in to your inner wisdom. You will discover how to create Vision Board Art as a *map to possibilities*, and unlock your potential creative energy. It is a simple and fun adventure that can also be a tool to help you manifest your goals and dreams.

Many of my clients are creative, innovative trendsetters, well-educated and yet still find they seem to come up against invisible roadblocks that hold them back from reaching their financial, health, or relationship objectives The key to success is communication, with others... and with *yourself*.

As a Certified ASR Educator, I will train you how to conceptualize your needs and desires through rational negotiation that overcomes emotional reaction, through one-on-one coaching and group sessions. Androgenous Semantic Realignment® (ASR) is the verbal communication theory developed by relationship counselor and therapist Dr. Pat Allen that improves understanding and facilitates positive communication in all your relationships, personal and business. It's an umbrella neurolinguistic framework that employs cognitive behavioral modification and is based on the latest scientific understanding of the differences in male and female mindsets which overarches my Vision Board Counseling and Personal Branding training systems for life success.

> **TESTIMONIAL:**
>
> Judith reached out to me and offered to create a visualization board for my garden design practice as well as new ventures I am planning. Judith's visualization boards are amazing, inspiring and display both insight and active elements that motivate people to "own their goals." I recommend Judith as mentor, collaborator and coordinator for any creative and literary projects.
>
> *Shirley Bovshow,*
> *Host of "Garden World Report"*

For more information about how you can use Vision Boards and Communication Training to set life goals and attain them, email me at *sarchjudith@gmail.com* **or call 323-455-4584 for a free consultation and discovery session.**

READER'S NOTES

Are You a Highly Sensitive Person?

- **Do you often get overwhelmed and crave "alone time"?**

- **Do you struggle with a heightened reaction to subtleties in your environment — sights, sounds, smells?**

- **Do you know a deep emotional appreciation of nature, music, art that other people seem to lack?**

- **Have you ever feared there might be something wrong because you feel and respond so differently from everyone you know?**

- **Have you ever been dissed that you're "too over-sensitive"?**

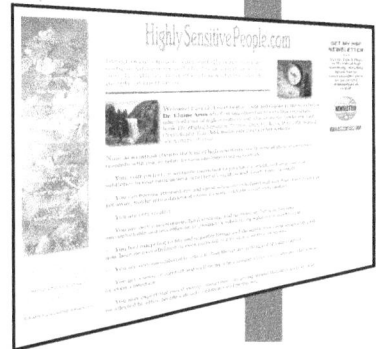

CONGRATULATIONS! There is **nothing wrong** with you.

You see, you have a special gift shared by less than 15% of men and women. I'm Jim Hallowes, and my website exploring the **Trait of High Sensitivity** has helped thousands of visitors like you who sometimes truly feel they were "born on another planet" come to terms with why their emotions, minds and bodies seem to somehow out of sync with everyone around them.

You need to know: You are gifted with a rare, inherited characteristic of your personality that puts you in a class shared by many very successful and accomplished people from Mozart and Michaelangelo to Steve Jobs. And once you discover how your brain and body work and understand the science that explains why you respond differently, you'll find that this special trait opens you up to **amazing potential**.

It has been said that, *"With great power comes great responsibility."*

To understand how your success in life will benefit from taking advantage of your sensitivities and protecting yourself and your gifts, and to understand your special relationship with others as their sensitive "priestly advisor" in a sometimes very insensitive world... make it a point to visit:

HighlySensitivePeople.com

www.ingramcontent.com/pod-product-compliance
Lightning Source LLC
Chambersburg PA
CBHW081229090426
42738CB00016B/3234